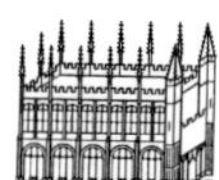

Minimally Invasive Spine Surgery: Advanced Surgical Techniques

System requirements: 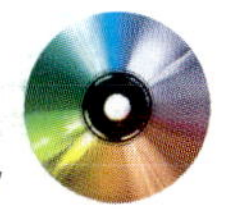

- **Operating System—Windows Vista or above**
- **Web Browser—Google Chrome, Mozilla Firefox, Internet Explorer 9 and above**
- **Essential plugins—Java & Flash Player**
  - If you are experiencing problems viewing content, please check that your system has Java enabled.
  - If the video clips do not appear, your system may require Flash Player or require an update to Flash Player settings. To learn more about Flash Player settings, please click on the link in the "Help" section of the DVD.
  - You can test Java and Flash Player by using the associated links available in the "Help" section of the DVD.

Please note that this CD/DVD will only play in a computer or laptop and will not work properly in a DVD player.

This CD/DVD come with an "Autorun" function; it may take a few seconds to load on your computer. If the content does not load, please follow the steps listed below to access the contents manually:

- Click on "My Computer".
- Select the CD/DVD drive and Click "Open/Explore". A list of available files will appear.
- Find and double click the file "launch.html".

For more information about troubleshooting, please click on http://support.microsoft.com/kb/330135.

Minimally Invasive Spine Surgery: Advanced Surgical Techniques

Editors

Kern Singh MD
Associate Professor
Co-Director, Minimally Invasive Spine Institute at Rush
Department of Orthopedic Surgery
Rush University Medical Center
Chicago, Illinois, USA

Alexander R Vaccaro MD PhD
Richard H Rothman Professor and Chairman
Department of Orthopedic Surgery
Professor of Neurosurgery
Co-Director, Delaware Valley Spinal Cord Injury Center
Co-Chief of Spine Surgery
Sidney Kimmel Medical Center at Thomas Jefferson University
President, Rothman Institute
Philadelphia, Pennsylvania, USA

Foreword

Frank M Phillips MD

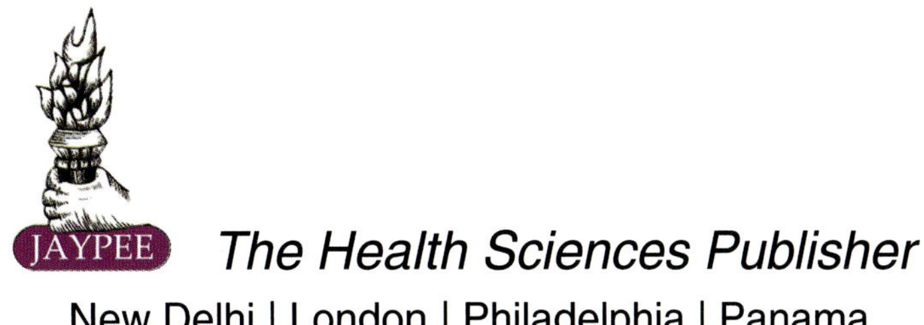

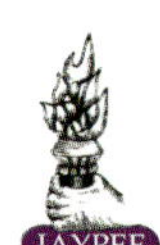

Jaypee Brothers Medical Publishers (P) Ltd

Headquarters
Jaypee Brothers Medical Publishers (P) Ltd.
4838/24, Ansari Road, Daryaganj
New Delhi 110 002, India
Phone: +91-11-43574357
Fax: +91-11-43574314
E-mail: jaypee@jaypeebrothers.com

Overseas Offices
J.P. Medical Ltd.
83, Victoria Street, London
SW1H 0HW (UK)
Phone: +44-20 3170 8910
Fax: +44(0)20 3008 6180
E-mail: info@jpmedpub.com

Jaypee-Highlights Medical Publishers Inc.
City of Knowledge, Bld. 237, Clayton
Panama City, Panama
Phone: +1 507-301-0496
Fax: +1 507-301-0499
E-mail: cservice@jphmedical.com

Jaypee Medical Inc.
The Bourse
111 South Independence Mall East
Suite 835
Philadelphia, PA 19106, USA
Phone: +1 267-519-9789
E-mail: jpmed.us@gmail.com

Jaypee Brothers Medical Publishers (P) Ltd.
17/1-B, Babar Road, Block-B, Shaymali
Mohammadpur, Dhaka-1207
Bangladesh
Mobile: +08801912003485
E-mail: jaypeedhaka@gmail.com

Jaypee Brothers Medical Publishers (P) Ltd.
Bhotahity, Kathmandu, Nepal
Phone: +977-9741283608
E-mail: kathmandu@jaypeebrothers.com

Website: www.jaypeebrothers.com
Website: www.jaypeedigital.com

Inquiries for bulk sales may be solicited at: jaypee@jaypeebrothers.com

Minimally Invasive Spine Surgery: Advanced Surgical Techniques

First Edition: 2016

ISBN: 978-93-5152-493-9

Printed at Ajanta Offset & Packagings Ltd., New Delhi

Dedicated to

My wife. Thank you for supporting me without question, being my closest friend when I need you most, and for helping me to raise our two children. I also dedicate this book to my two children, Suraj and Siya, you give me unbelievable joy every day of my life.

Kern Singh

The new addition to my family: Christian John Vaccaro, born January 22nd, 2015. His life is a continuous source of joy for the entire family.

Alexander R Vaccaro

Contributors

Junyoung Ahn
Clinical Research Coordinator
Department of Orthopedic Surgery
Rush University Medical Center
Chicago, Illinois, USA

Neel Anand MD
Clinical Professor of Surgery
Department of Orthopedic Surgery
Cedars-Sinai Medical Center
Los Angeles, California, USA

Daniel D Bohl MD MPH
Resident
Department of Orthopedic Surgery
Rush University Medical Center
Chicago, Illinois, USA

Thomas D Cha MD MBA
Instructor
Department of Orthopedic Surgery
Massachusetts General Hospital
Boston, Massachusetts, USA

Gabriel Duhancioglu MS
Research Assistant
Department of Orthopedic Surgery
Rush University Medical Center
Chicago, Illinois, USA

Hamid Hassanzadeh MD
Assistant Professor
Department of Orthopedic Surgery
University of Virginia
Charlottesville, Virginia, USA

Rahul Kamath MS
Research Assistant
Department of Orthopedic Surgery
Rush University Medical Center
Chicago, Illinois, USA

Safdar N Khan MD
Associate Professor
Department of Orthopedics
The Ohio State University
Columbus, Ohio, USA

Mark F Kurd MD
Assistant Professor
Department of Orthopedic Surgery
The Rothman Institute
Thomas Jefferson University
Philadelphia, Pennsylvania, USA

Damandeep Singh Makkar DNB(Ortho)
Chief Spine Surgeon
Department of Orthopedics and
Spine Surgery
Arora Neuro Center
Ludhiana, Punjab, India

Alejandro Marquez-Lara MD
Research Fellow
Department of Orthopedic Surgery
Rush University Medical Center
Chicago, Illinois, USA

Sreeharsha V Nandyala
Research Fellow
Department of Orthopedics
Rush University Medical Center
Chicago, Illinois, USA

Daniel K Park MD
Assistant Professor
Department of Orthopedics
William Beaumont Hospital
Royal Oak, Michigan, USA

Alpesh A Patel MD
Associate Professor
Department of Orthopedics
Northwestern University
Chicago, Illinois, USA

Sheeraz A Qureshi MD
Associate Professor
Orthopedic Surgeon
Department of Orthopedic Surgery
Icahn School of Medicine at
Mount Sinai
New York, New York, USA

Kris B Siemionow MD
Chief of Spine Surgery
Assistant Professor of Orthopedics
and Neurosurgery
University of Illinois
Chicago, Illinois, USA

Kern Singh MD
Associate Professor
Co-Director, Minimally Invasive
Spine Institute at Rush
Department of Orthopedic Surgery
Rush University Medical Center
Chicago, Illinois, USA

Branko Skovrlj MD
Resident
Department of Neurosurgery
Icahn School of Medicine at
Mount Sinai
New York, New York, USA

Alexander R Vaccaro MD PhD
Richard H Rothman Professor and
Chairman
Department of Orthopedic Surgery
Professor of Neurosurgery
Co-Director, Delaware Valley Spinal
Cord Injury Center
Co-Chief of Spine Surgery
Sidney Kimmel Medical Center at
Thomas Jefferson University
President, Rothman Institute
Philadelphia, Pennsylvania, USA

Foreword

The goals of any patient undergoing spinal surgery are to realize an excellent clinical outcome with a low risk of complications, minimal peri-operative pain or discomfort and rapid resumption of normal activities. In the past with open spine surgery, certain of these goals were often achieved at the expense of another. As enabling technologies have evolved over the last decades, all of these surgical goals can now be achieved with less invasive surgical techniques. Minimally invasive spine (MIS) surgery has become far more predictable and reproducible and the data supporting these approaches has expanded. As MIS surgical approaches are developed, the challenge of appropriately educating surgeons to achieve proficiency in these techniques is substantial. Open surgical skills do not necessarily translate into MIS skills and a difficult learning curve putting our patients at risk is unacceptable.

Drs Singh and Vaccaro have compiled an outstanding text, guiding the reader and viewer through surgical indications, pertinent anatomy, set-up and techniques in an easy to follow sequence. Although brief, each chapter does an outstanding job of succinctly capturing the essence of the procedure and associated pitfalls. The consistency between chapters makes the book easy to follow. This text should serve as a useful resource for both trainees and the experienced spine surgeon. In addition, its value as an overview and reference before performing a procedure cannot be underestimated.

Frank M Phillips MD
Professor, Orthopedic Surgery
Spine Fellowship Co-Director
Rush University Medical Center
Chicago, Illinois, USA

Preface

Minimally invasive spine surgery has gained significant interest due to the reported expedited postoperative recovery, decreased blood loss, shorter length of hospital stay, and lower postoperative pain as compared to the traditional open techniques. Through carefully curated figures, radiographs, and commentary, this book describes the innovative techniques, evidence, and controversies surrounding minimally invasive spine surgery. We believe that orthopedic surgeons, neurosurgeons, and surgical trainees, such as students, residents, and fellows, will benefit from the step-by-step descriptions of the techniques in both the text and the narrated video demonstrations.

Kern Singh
Alexander R Vaccaro

Acknowledgments

I would like to personally thank Steve Fineberg, Alejandro Marquez-Lara, Sreeharsha Nandyala, and Junyoung Ahn for all their tireless hard work on this book. Every individual on this list has made me proud of what they have accomplished and what they will accomplish as they begin their careers in orthopedic surgery.

I would also like to thank the Senior Management team and Production staff of Jaypee Brothers Medical Publishers (P) in Philadelphia and in New Delhi, India.

Kern Singh

Contents

Video Legends

1. Minimally Invasive Percutaneous Dilation
2. Minimally Invasive Posterior Cervical Foraminotomy
3. Percutaneous Pedicle Screw Placement
4. Kyphoplasty–Percutaneous Cement Augmentation
5. Minimally Invasive Lumbar Discectomy (LD)
6. Minimally Invasive Transforaminal Lumbar Interbody Fusion (TLIF)
7. Minimally Invasive Lateral Lumbar Interbody Fusion (LLIF)
8. Mini-Open Anterior Lumbar Interbody Fusion (ALIF)
9. Mini-Open Lateral Lumbar Corpectomy
10. Minimally Invasive Far Lateral Lumbar Discectomy
11. Minimally Invasive Thoracic Corpectomy

Chapter 1

Introduction to Minimally Invasive Spine Surgery

Kern Singh, Alejandro Marquez-Lara, Sreeharsha V Nandyala, Alexander R Vaccaro

INTRODUCTION

Minimally invasive spine surgery (MISS) has gained considerable momentum as growing evidence suggests comparable clinical outcomes as well as less postoperative morbidity and faster patient recovery than conventional open surgery. Since the inception of MISS in the late 1970s, significant advancements in instrumentation, imaging modalities, and surgical techniques have improved visualization, guidance, and enabled surgeons to address a wide spectrum of spinal pathology while sparing important soft tissue structures.

PRINCIPLES AND PATIENT SELECTION FOR MISS

Basic Principles[1]

- Preservation of anatomic structures
  - Anatomic neurovascular and muscular planes are utilized to access the spine.
    - An intermuscular working plane (Wiltse plane) (Fig. 1.1) is developed utilizing blunt sequential dilators (Fig. 1.2) that minimize tissue injury thereby reducing postoperative pain.
    - Narrow self-retaining retractors provide a steady visual field while avoiding excessive muscle retraction (Fig. 1.3).
  - The tendon attachment sites of key muscles (e.g. multifidus) are preserved with MISS. This anatomic approach reduces the potential risk for muscle denervation and postoperative paraspinal muscle weakness.
- Surgical feasibility
  - MISS techniques aim to avoid important anatomic structures (e.g. neural structures, great vessels) that are traditionally at risk with open surgery.
    - Precise knowledge of the patient's anatomy and the utilization of neuromonitoring devices (e.g. continuous electromyographic stimulation) can prevent injury to vital structures.
  - Surgical magnification (microscope or loupes) enable detailed identification of critical neurovascular structures for safe manipulation and dissection.

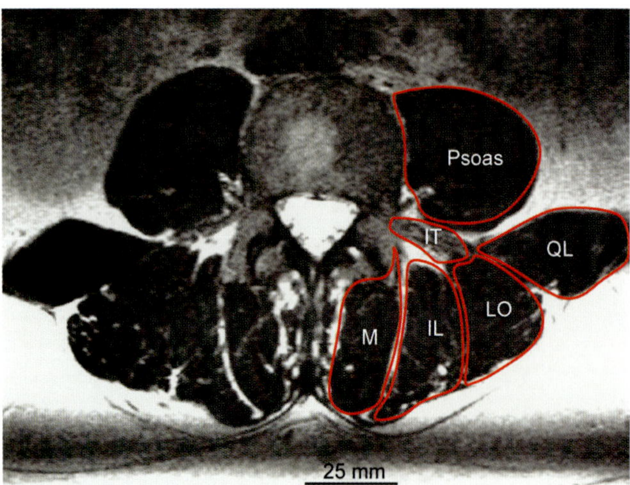

Fig. 1.1: Magnetic resonance imaging cross-section of the L4-L5 disc space highlighting the paraspinal muscles: multifidus (M), iliocostalis (IL) longissimus (LO), quadratus lumborum (QL), intertransversarii (IT), and psoas muscles.[1]

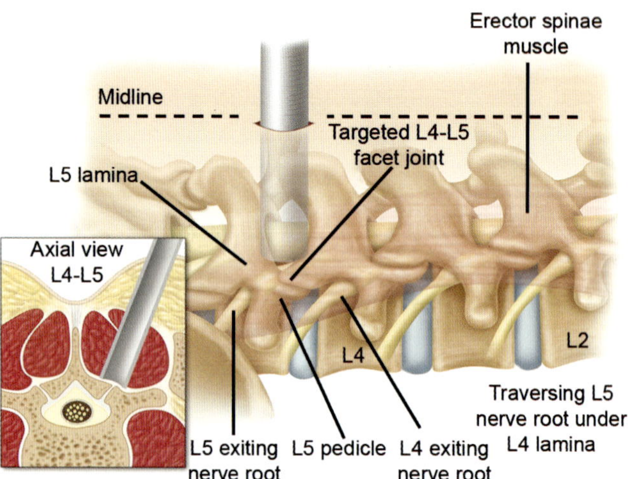

Fig. 1.2: Blunt sequential dilators are utilized to create an intermuscular surgical working channel and minimize soft tissue injury.

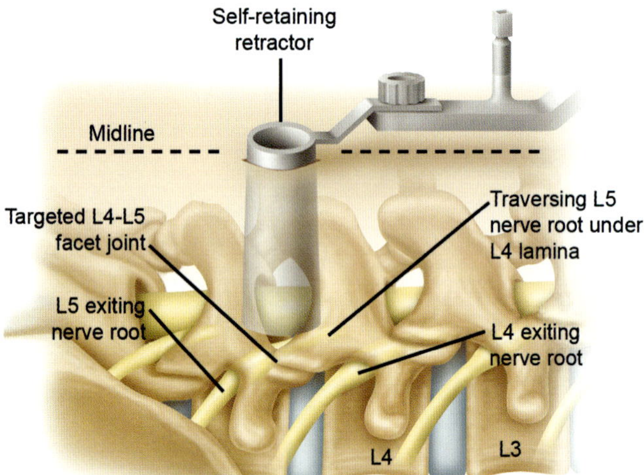

Fig. 1.3: A self-retaining retractor is fixed in place with a table mounted arm.

- Awareness of the patient's three-dimensional bony anatomy and its correlation to the two-dimensional radiographic imaging will help guide the trajectory and depth of the instruments utilized in MISS (Figs. 1.4A to C).

Factors Affecting Patient Selection in MISS

- Clinical presentation—Similar to the success of an open procedure, patient selection remains the mainstay of ensuring excellent clinical outcomes after MISS.
- Obesity—The girth of the surrounding soft tissue may limit the utilization of open surgical retractors. However, obese patients may benefit the most from an MISS procedure.

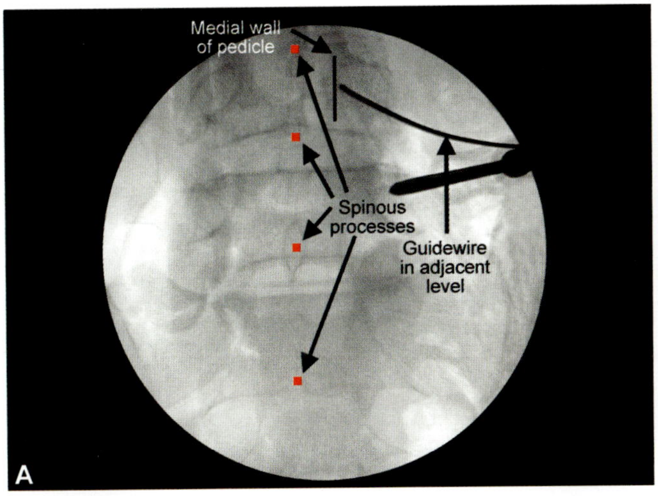

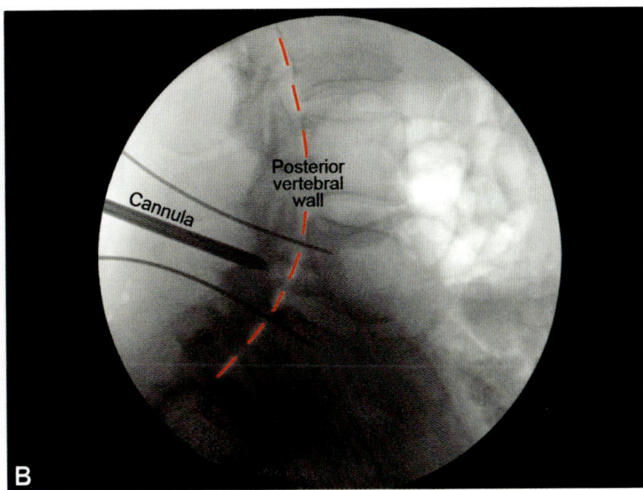

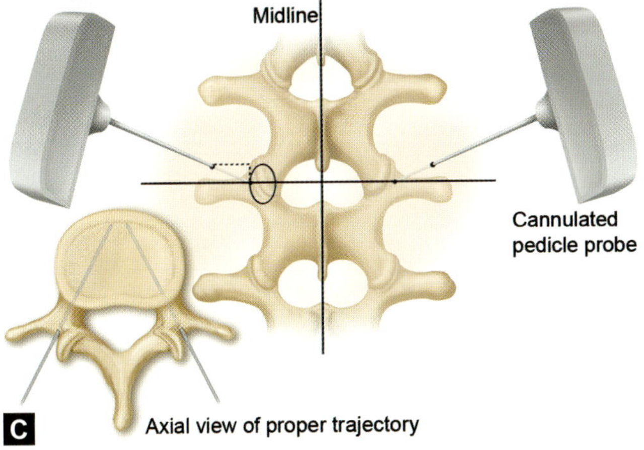

Figs. 1.4A to C: (A) Anteroposterior intraoperative fluoroscopic image demarcating important anatomical landmarks (e.g. spinous process, medial wall of the pedicle). (B) Lateral intraoperative fluoroscopic image delineating the posterior vertebral wall. (C) Cannulated pedicle probes placed in the correct orientation and depth for cement augmentation.

- Revision surgery—Previously altered anatomy and scar tissue pose a significant challenge for a minimally invasive approach. Although feasible, this should be reserved for surgeons with ample experience with MISS techniques.
- Surgical learning curve—The number of cases required to become proficient is dependent upon the technical skill of the surgeon and complexity of the procedure.
- Complexity of the procedure—Minimally invasive techniques have been developed to address multilevel cases with or without deformity. However, these cases should only be attempted by experienced surgeons.

ANATOMIC AND PHYSIOLOGIC CONSIDERATIONS WITH MISS

Paraspinal Muscles

- Deep paramedian transversospinalis muscles
  - Multifidus
    - The multifidus is the most important posterior stabilizer of the spine.

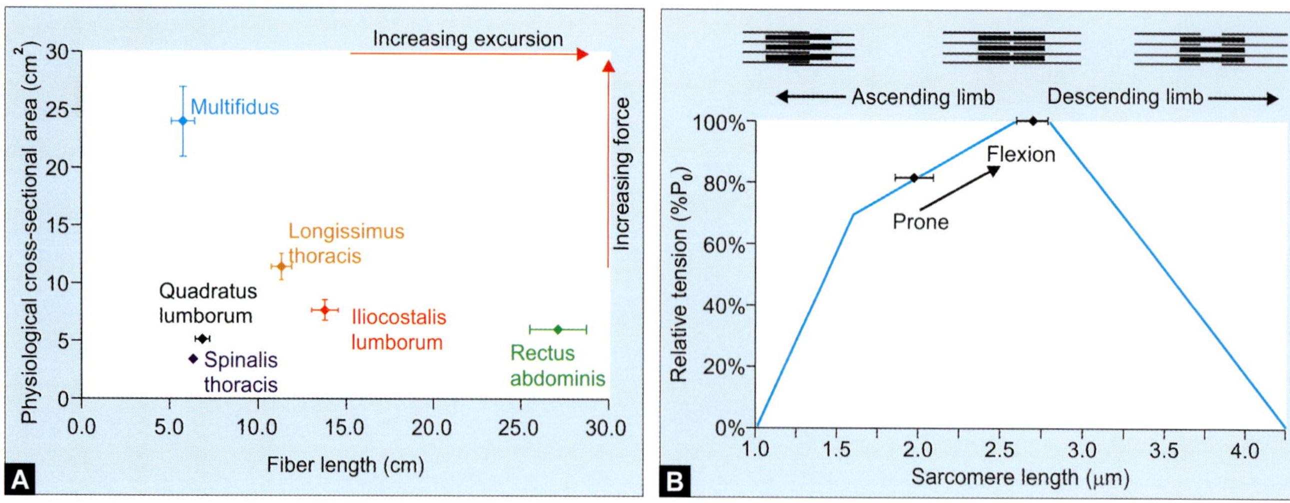

Figs. 1.5A and B: (A) A scatter plot of the physiological cross-sectional area versus fiber length, which illustrates the functional design of the paraspinal muscles. The data demonstrate that the multifidus has the largest force generating capacity in the lumbar spine (B) The sarcomere length operating range of the multifidus plotted on the human skeletal muscle sarcomere length tension curve (black line).[1]

- Multiple separate fasciculi are characteristic of the multifidus muscle. Each fasciculus originates from the transverse process of the corresponding vertebrae and inserts into the spinous process of the cephalad vertebrae 1–4 levels above its origin.
- This unique structure provides a large physiologic cross-sectional area that enables the multifidus to create large forces over short distances.
- At rest, each sarcomere is positioned along the ascending portion of the length-tension curve (Figs. 1.5A and B).
  - This physiologic quality enables the multifidus to produce greater force as the spine flexes forward at its most vulnerable position.
- Superficial and lateral erector spinae muscles
  - Longissimus
    - The muscle fibers originate from the transverse and accessory processes and insert distally into the ventral surface of the posterior superior iliac spine.
  - Iliocostalis
    - The muscle fibers originate from the tip of the transverse processes and adjacent thoracolumbar fascia and insert distally into the ventral edge of the iliac crest.
  - The longissimus and iliocostalis muscles run lateral to the multifidus, contain longer muscle fibers, and have a relatively small cross-sectional area. As such, they function to extend, rotate, and bend the trunk.

The Sequelae of Open Surgery

- Posterior midline approaches to the lumbar spine can potentiate muscle atrophy.
  - The multifidus is most likely to be injured with an open approach.
    - This disruption of the multifidus can compromise the dynamic stability of the spine and delay patient recovery.

- Physiological events that potentiate muscle atrophy
  - Direct muscle injury
  - The utilization of powerful self-retaining retractors creates areas of ischemia. Depending upon the procedural time and the amount of force against the soft tissue, permanent damage may result.
- In addition, once the retractors are released, the remaining muscle fibers are prone to reperfusion injury.
  - Muscle denervation
  - The multifidus receives a monosegmental innervation from the medial branch nerve that originates from the dorsal rami of each lumbar spinal nerve.
  - The monosegmental innervation leaves the muscle particularly vulnerable to injury.
- If the latissimus and iliocostalis muscles are injured, postoperative extension strength can be significantly compromised.

HOSPITAL COSTS ASSOCIATED WITH MISS

- Direct costs[2,3]
  - Blood bank costs
    - MISS procedures are associated with less blood loss and blood transfusion volume.
    - Standard type and cross-match studies are done on a case-by-case basis and are rarely done with elective MISS procedures.
  - Pharmacy costs
    - Smaller incisions and less soft tissue damage associated with minimally invasive procedures will result in less postoperative pain and narcotic requirements.
  - Room and board (length of stay)
    - The shorter hospital stay after a minimally invasive procedure will reduce hospital resource utilization.
  - Surgical service costs
    - The procedural and anesthesia times are significantly reduced with minimally invasive techniques.
  - Implant costs
    - In both open and MISS techniques, the cost of implants contributes to the majority of the total direct costs.
- Indirect costs
  - Postoperative complications
    - A less invasive surgical approach has been associated with fewer postoperative complications including surgical site infections.
  - Discharge disposition
    - Less postoperative pain enables participation in outpatient rehabilitation and may potentiate a faster recovery.
  - Reoperation and revision procedures
    - MISS has demonstrated lower reoperation rates when compared with open techniques in the early postoperative period.
    - However, there is limited data regarding the long-term outcomes associated with minimally invasive techniques.

Pearls

- Hospitals may consider the reduced operative time, hospital stay, and blood transfusion requirements associated with minimally invasive techniques as an opportunity to increase surgical volume.

- Missed days of work
  - Less postoperative pain and a faster recovery after MISS may enable the patient to return to work sooner when compared with an open procedure.

ANESTHESIA TECHNIQUES AND POSTOPERATIVE ANALGESIA IN MISS[4]

Preoperative Considerations

- Patients with a history of chronic opioid dependence may benefit from a preoperative evaluation by a pain specialist.
- Screening for obstructive sleep apnea (OSA) is important to determine if patients are amenable to a fast-track postoperative pain protocol.
  - Postoperative opioids may cause significant respiratory collapse in patients with OSA.
- A combination of nonsteroidal anti-inflammatory drugs (NSAIDs) and sustained release opioids can be initiated 2–3 days prior to the procedure.
  - This enables the accumulation of medication to suppress the inflammatory response associated with the surgical procedure (e.g. prostaglandin E_2).
- Preoperative analgesics (day of surgery)
  - High-dose NSAIDs (e.g. 400 mg of celecoxib) orally
    - In the case of fusion surgeries, this is not recommended.
  - Acetaminophen (1000 mg)
  - Sustained release oxycodone (10–20 mg).
  - Other pain medications that may benefit patients include:
    - Gabapentin (600 mg)
    - Pregabalin (100–150 mg)
- Nonanalgesic medication
  - IV fluid administrated may reduce perioperative nausea, dizziness, and drowsiness.
  - Antiemetics
    - 5-HT3 blockers (ondansetron 4 mg IV)
    - Scopolamine patch

Intraoperative Anesthesia

- General anesthesia
  - Induction—Propofol
  - Maintenance—Sevoflurane or desflurane
  - IV opioids—Sufentanil or remifentanil
    - IV opioids provide a steady state of anesthesia.
- Anesthesia effect on neurophysiological monitoring [somatosensory-evoked potentials (SSEP)].
  - Inhalation agents can reduce the amplitude and latency of SSEP signals.
  - Alternate analgesics (short-acting opioids) may be preferred.

Pearls

- Monitored anesthesia care (MAC) may be adequate for single level procedures with an estimated surgical time of 30-90 minutes.
- Liberal use of local anesthetic is recommended.

- Local anesthetic
  - Generous infiltration of lidocaine 1% in the surgical incision site is recommended as it will reduce the patient's analgesic requirements.
  - Deep tissue should be infiltrated with bupivacaine 0.25%.
    - Care must be taken to assure the anesthetic does not spread to the nerve roots, as this can obscure neurologic assessment postoperatively.
- Other medications
  - IV fluids and vasopressors as needed to minimize hypotension.
  - Antiemetics (5-HT3 blockers)

Postoperative Analgesia

- NSAIDs should be continued for 2 weeks after surgery.
  - NSAIDs should not be utilized after spinal fusion procedures.
- Sustained release oxycodone is continued in the postoperative period.
- Muscle relaxants (tizanidine or baclofen) will address muscle spasms related to the surgical intervention.
- Gabapentinoids (gabapentin and pregabalin) can be utilized depending upon the extent of the surgical trauma.

Pitfalls

- Sedation from the combination of opioids and gabapentin may significantly delay initiation of therapy.

REFERENCES

1. Kim CW. Scientific basis of minimally invasive spine surgery—prevention of multifidus muscle injury during posterior lumbar surgery. Spine 2010;35: S281-6.
2. Lucio JC, Vanconia RB, Deluzio KJ, et al. Economics of less invasive spinal surgery: an analysis of hospital cost differences between open and minimally invasive instrumented spinal fusion procedures during the perioperative period. Risk Manag Healthcare Policy 2012;5:65-74.
3. Wang MY, Lerner J, Lesko J, McGirt MJ. Acute hospital costs after minimally invasive versus open lumbar interbody fusion—data from a US national database with 6106 patients. J Spinal Disord Tech. 2012;25:324-8.
4. Buvanendran A, Thillainathan V. Preoperative and postoperative anesthetic and analgesic techniques for minimally invasive surgery of the spine. Spine 2010;35:S274-80.

REFERENCE SUMMARY

1. Kim CW. Scientific Basis of Minimally Invasive Spine Surgery—Prevention of multifidus muscle injury during posterior lumbar surgery. Spine 2010;35: S281-S286.
   Summary: A literature review describing the paraspinal musculature along with the structure, insertion, innervation, and function. The authors report the significant anatomic and physiologic consequences of disturbing these structures with an open spinal procedure.
2. Lucio JC, Vanconia RB, Deluzio KJ, Lehmen JA, Rodgers JA, Rodgers W. Economics of less invasive spinal surgery: an analysis of hospital cost differences between open and minimally invasive instrumented spinal fusion procedures during the perioperative period. Risk Management and Healthcare Policy 2012;5:65-74.
   Summary: A retrospective review comparing the costs associated with 101 open posterior lumbar fusions and 109 minimally invasive procedures. The authors report an average cost savings of $2825 with MIS procedures. In addition, the authors noted significantly less blood loss, shorter hospital stay, and lower complication rates in the MIS cohort.

3. Wang MY, Lerner J, Lesko J, McGirt MJ. Acute hospital costs after minimally invasive versus open lumbar interbody fusion- data from a US national database with 6106 patients. J Spinal Disord Tech 2012;25:324-328.
Summary: A retrospective analysis of hospital charges, length of stay, and dicharge disposition in 74 patients treated with 1- and 2-level MIS and open posterior lumbar fusions. The authors reported that MIS procedures resulted in a shorter hospital stay, reduced hospital charges, and lower transfer rates to inpatient rehabilitation centers.
4. Buvanendran A, Thillainathan V. Preoperative and postoperative anesthetic and analgesic techniques for minimally invasive surgery of the Spine. Spine 2010;35:S274-S280
Summary: A literature review of the current anesthesia and analgesia protocols utilized in minimally invasive spine surgery. The authors highlight the literature supporting the utilization of multimodal analgesic therapy with a fast-track anaesthesia with MISS.

Chapter

2

Retractor Systems in Minimally Invasive Spine Surgery

Sreeharsha V Nandyala, Mark F Kurd, Kern Singh

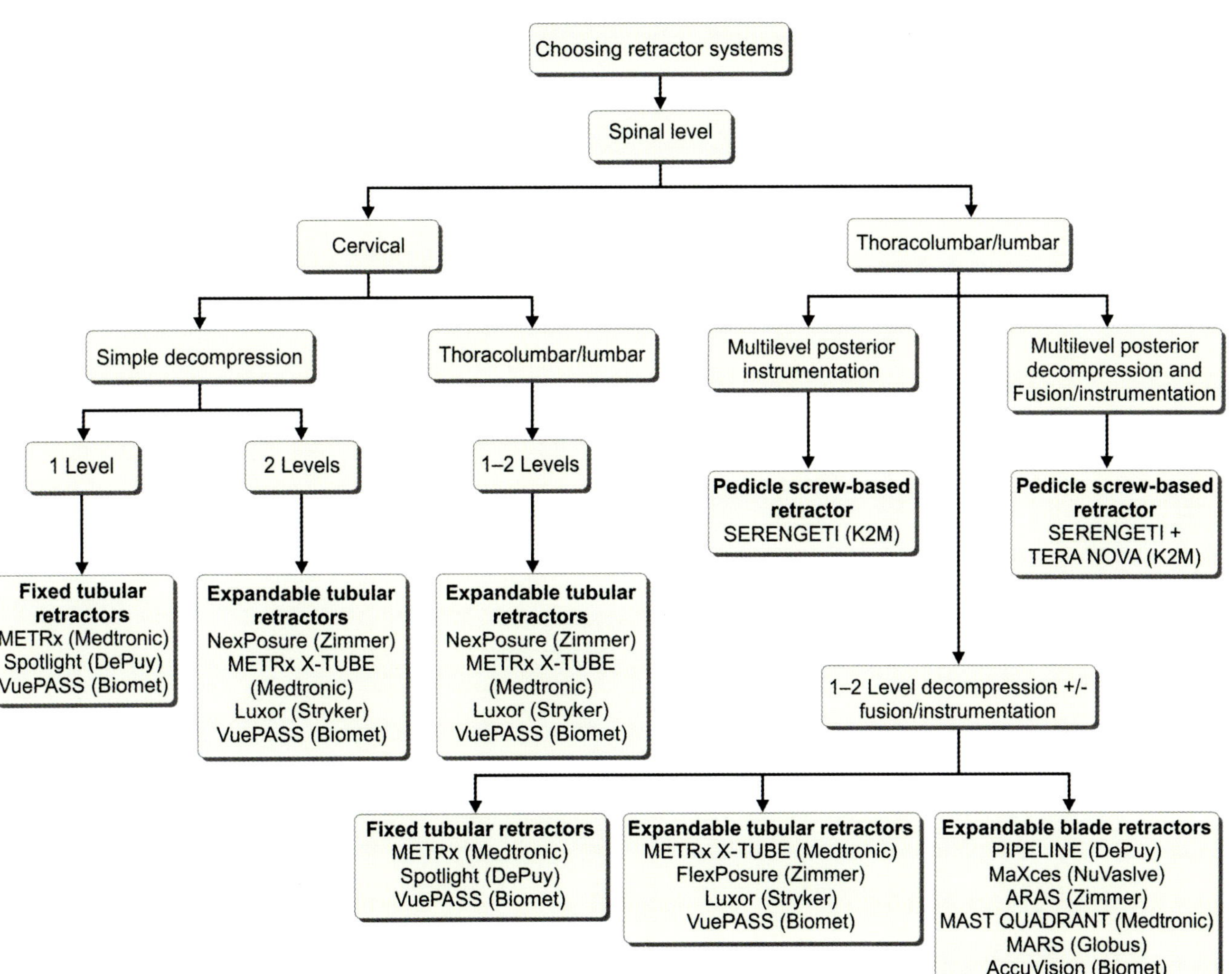

ANATOMIC CONSIDERATIONS

- The posterior cervical fascia (superficial/investing and prevertebral) is thicker than the thoracolumbar fascia. A fasciotomy is particularly important in the cervical spine to allow easy passage of the instruments through the paraspinal muscles.

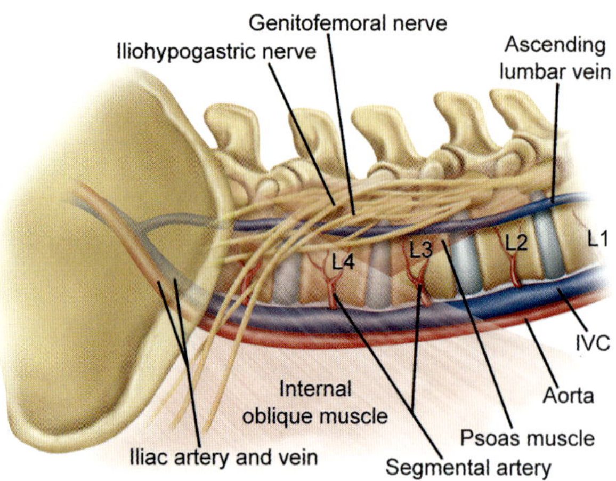

Fig. 2.1: The nerve structures forming the lumbar plexus traverse the lower lumbar levels, which limit the surgical "safe zone."

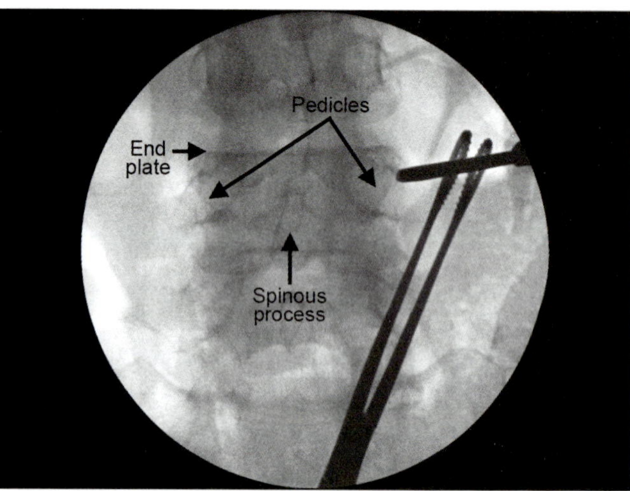

Fig. 2.2: Intraoperative fluoroscopic image demonstrating a true anteroposterior view. The spinous processes are at the midline, equidistant to the pedicles bilaterally.

- The three major lumbar paraspinal muscles are the multifidus, iliocostalis, and longissimus. These muscles provide dynamic and static stabilization of the thoracolumbar spine.
  - The multifidus is the most important of the paraspinal muscles due to its unique design and insertion pattern. The proximal fibers insert on the spinous process of the thoracolumbar vertebrae and attach distally on the transverse process of the caudal two to five adjacent vertebrae. Significant disruption to these insertion points can alter the stability of the spine.
- The lumbar plexus courses more ventral at the distal lumbar segments (L4–L5) when compared with the proximal segments. Thus, a lateral approach to the L4–L5 level represents the greatest risk for injury to the neural structures of the lumbar plexus (Fig. 2.1). Careful placement of the initial guidewire and dilator between the middle and anterior third of the vertebral body is crucial. In addition, retractors with integrated neuromonitoring enable real-time feedback.

Minimally Invasive Access

- The key to a successful and safe procedure relies upon proper patient positioning, adequate radiographic visualization of the anatomic landmarks, and a correct surgical incision site.
  - Patient position
    - Patient position will vary based upon the surgical intervention. Care must be taken to secure the patient on the bed. Adequately pad all bony prominences and position the arms anterior to the midline coronal axis of the body with <90° of shoulder abduction and >90° of elbow flexion.
    - If the patient position is altered during the procedure, the surgical field can become compromised.
  - Radiographic anatomic landmarks
    - The spinous processes should be in the midline of an anteroposterior radiograph (Fig. 2.2).

Pearls

- The initial dilator can often be utilized as an elevator with gentle subperiosteal dissection to sweep the paraspinal muscles off the lamina. Beginning medially on the spinous process and coursing lateral to the lamina may be beneficial.
- On occasion it may be necessary to sweep the psoas muscle posteriorly to safely dock the tube without nerve penetration.

Pitfalls

- Surgeons may experience difficulty in locating anatomic landmarks with the initial dilators. As such, care should be taken such that inadvertent interlaminar penetration does not occur.
- Sustained compression of the lumbar plexus against the transverse process may lead to a neurologic deficit. Minimizing retraction time and pressure during a lateral approach is essential.

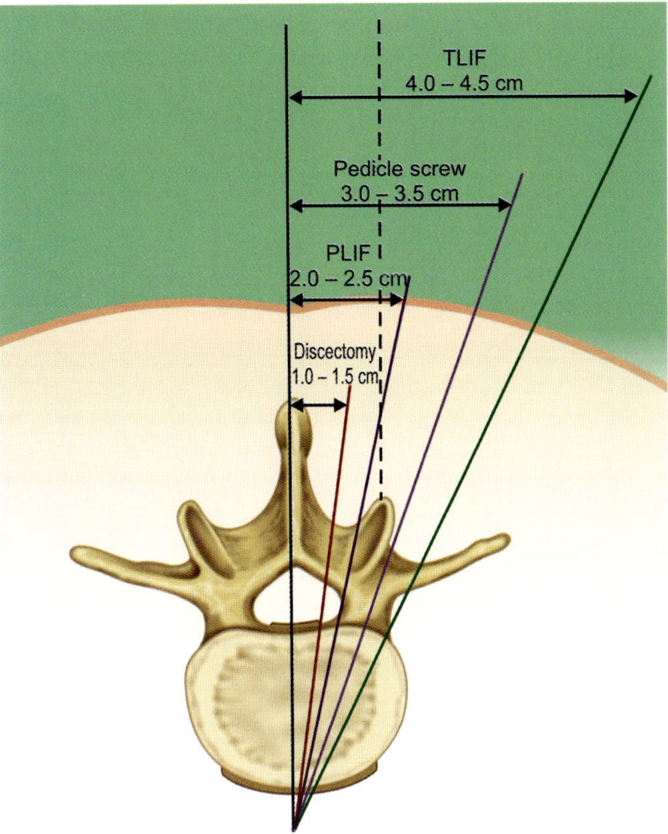

Fig. 2.3: Illustration demonstrating incision planning for various minimally invasive procedures. Modified with permission from Medtronic, Minneapolis, MN.

- The pedicles should lie equidistant to the spinous process on either side and the medial edge of the pedicle should be clearly identified.

- Surgical incision (Fig. 2.3)
  - Size: The size of the final working portal will determine the size of the incision (15–26 mm).
  - Incision site:
    - Discectomies
      - Paramedian: 5–10 mm from the midline
      - Far lateral: 30–40 mm from the midline
    - Laminectomies: 10–15 mm from the midline
    - Fusions: Lateral to the midpedicular line (20–25mm from the midline).
- Following a fasciotomy of the same length and inline with the skin incision, the initial dilator is placed through the paraspinal muscles, creating a Wiltse-type interval. Using the initial dilator, the spinous process can be palpated in the midline and then coursed lateral to palpate the lamina-facet junction. In the lumbar spine, the dilator should be docked on the caudal aspect of the cranial lamina. This allows access to the pars, lamina, and facet complex at the level of interest (Figs. 2.4A and B).

Pitfalls:

- Care must be taken to avoid plunging into the spinal canal during docking of the initial dilator.

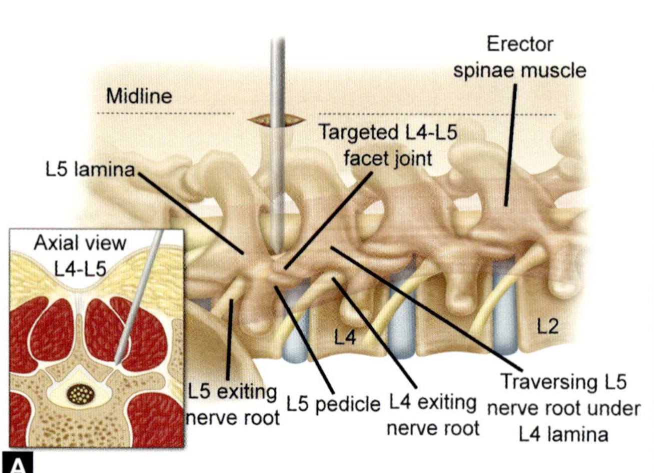

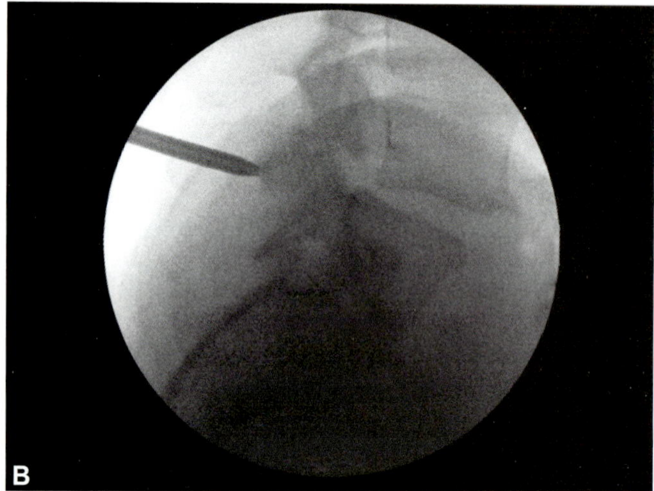

Figs. 2.4A and B: An initial dilator (A) is utilized to localize the disc space and create an intermuscular interval under fluoroscopic guidance (B).

- Sequential dilators are utilized to increase the working portal. Once the final dilator is placed, a final working portal is docked and firmly attached to the table-mounted arm (Figs. 2.5A to D).
  - The retractor arm should be mounted on the contralateral side of the surgeon to avoid obstruction of the operative field.
- A lateral fluoroscopic image should always be obtained to confirm appropriate localization at the level of interest.
- Once the retractor's position is confirmed, the surgical microscope can be brought into position.
  - Alternatively, surgical loupes may be utilized.
  - A light source may also be attached to the retractor arm, or the surgeon may wear a headlight to enhance visualization.

TYPES OF RETRACTORS

Nonexpandable Tubular Retractors (Figs. 2.6A and B)

- Design purpose
  - Microdecompression (cervical or lumbar)
  - Single-level fusion
- Design characteristics
  - A thin wall cylinder enables the retractor to withstand placement into deep surgical wounds. An arm extends from the superficial part of the retractor to attach to the table-mounted arm.
  - If well positioned, a retractor will define the necessary working corridor and prevent paraspinal muscles or soft tissue intrusion (creep) into the surgical field.
  - The cylinder can be circular or oval. The oval design maximizes cranial-caudal exposure to facilitate instrumentation while minimizing medial to lateral soft tissue compromise.

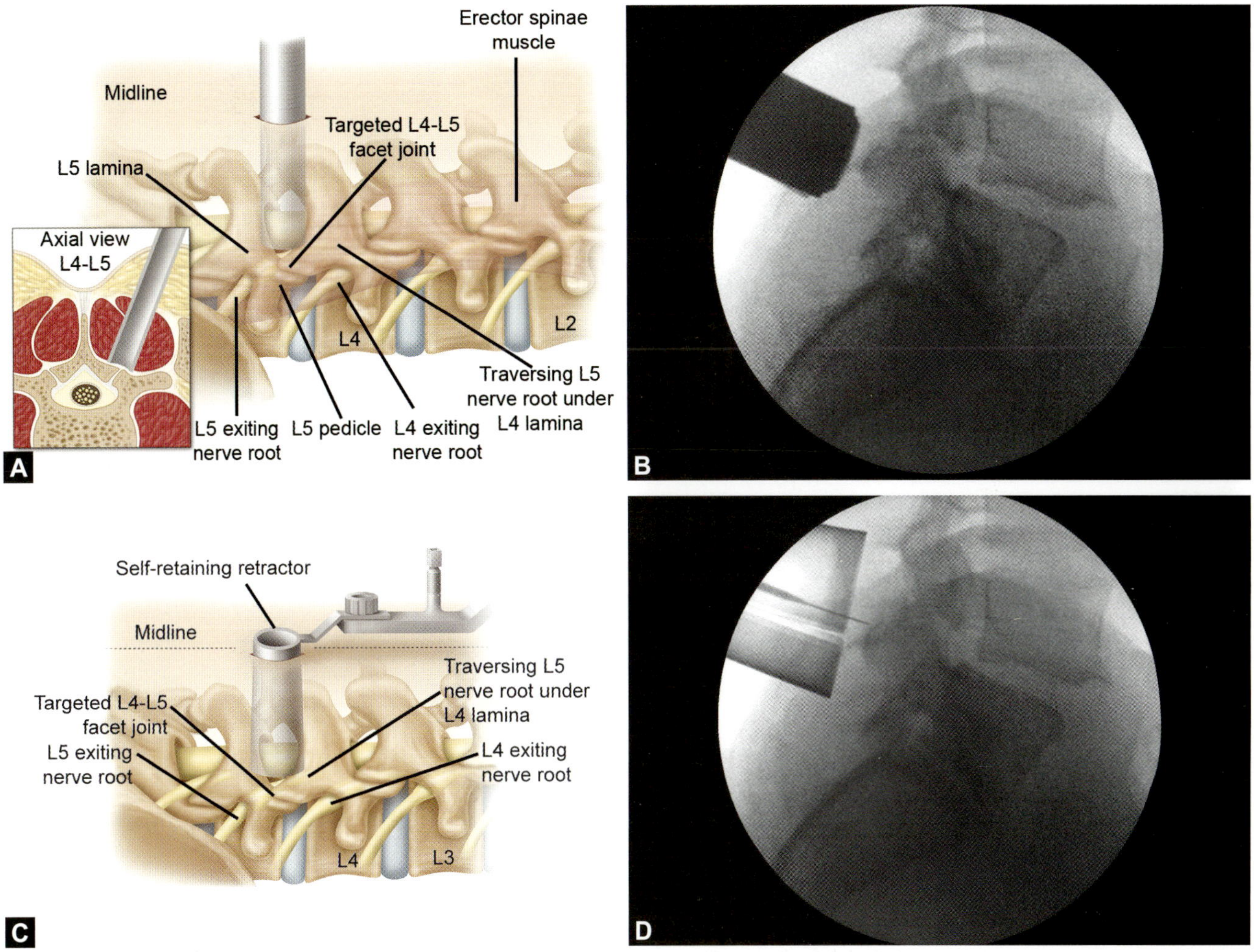

Figs. 2.5A to D: Sequential dilators (A) are utilized to increase the size of the working canal. After the final dilator is placed, intraoperative fluoroscopy confirms its position (B). A mounted retractor arm holds the surgical retractor in place (C) and a final X-ray is taken to confirm that the retractor is correctly positioned over the involved disc space (D).

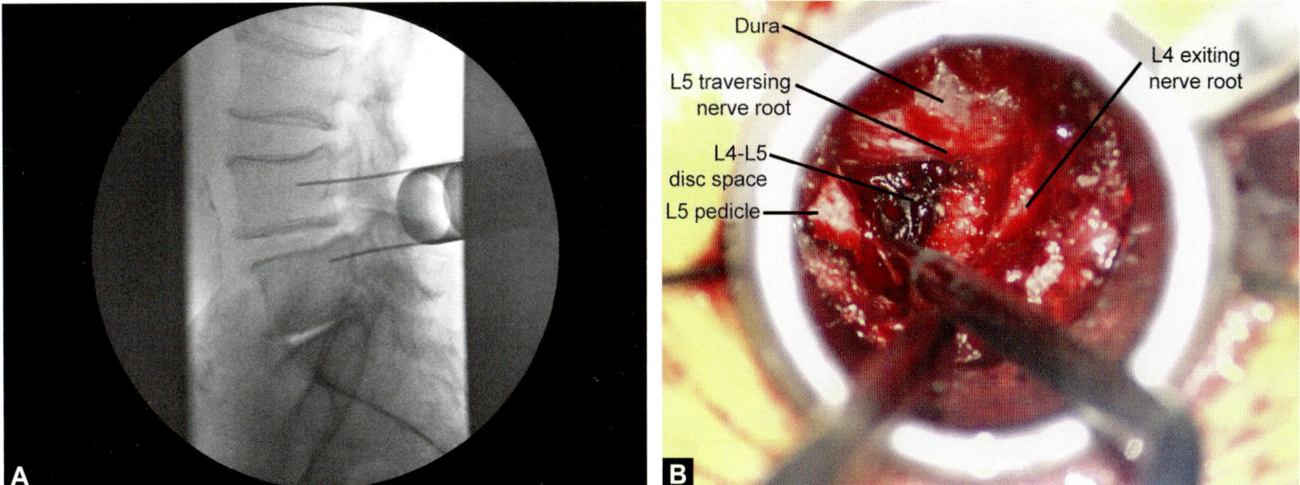

Figs. 2.6A and B: An example of a nonexpandable tubular retractor utilized during a transforaminal lumbar interbody fusion. Intraoperative radiograph (A) and working channel (B).

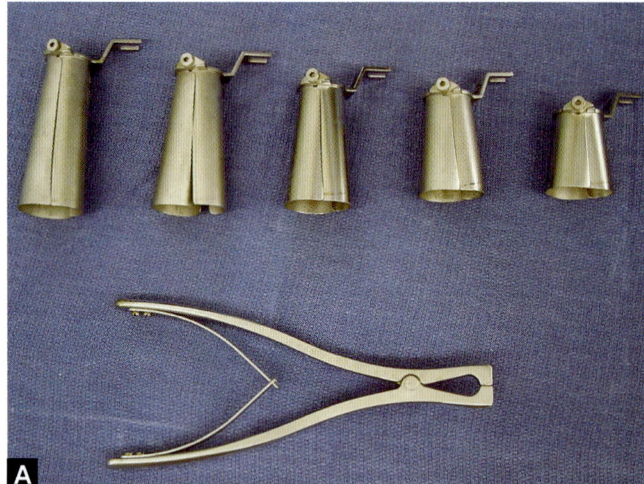

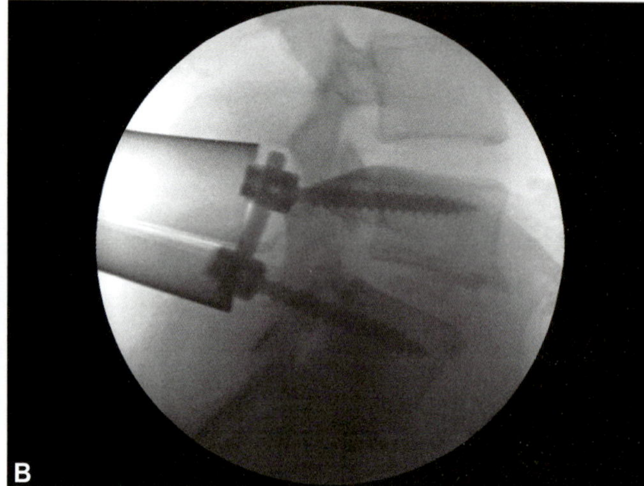

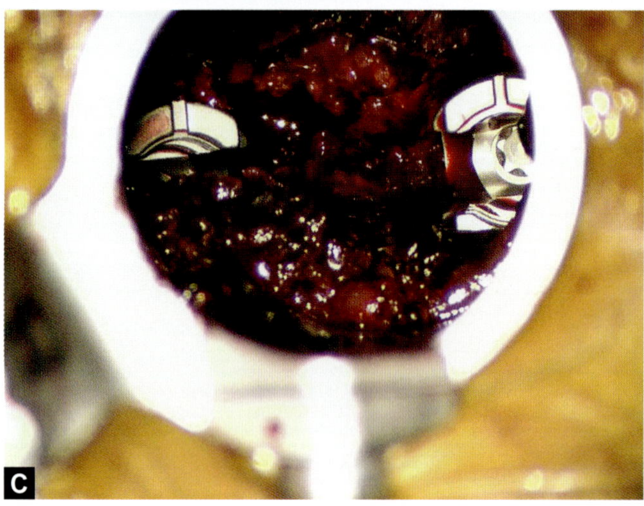

Figs. 2.7A to C: (A) Expandable retractors of various sizes. (B) An intraoperative lateral radiograph depicting the distal expansion of an expandable tubular retractor to increase the exposure and visualization. (C) Intraoperative photograph demonstrating the placement of pedicle screws under direct visualization through an expandable tubular retractor.

    - Alternatively a "wanding" technique (tilting the retractor to obtain a more favorable approach angle) can be utilized with a circular cylinder to increase surgical exposure.
  - Surgical anatomy can be visualized with surgical loupes or microscope magnification.
- Design limitations
  - The static nature of a nonexpandable retractor limits the amount of angulation that can be used to adapt to variations in the local anatomy.
  - The static long and narrow working corridor requires the utilization of specialized instruments and a unique level of manual dexterity. Retractor length always should be minimized to allow for the shortest working distance.

Expandable Tubular Retractors (Figs. 2.7A to C)

- Design purpose
  - 1–2 level fusions
  - Adjacent level pedicle screw placement

Pearl

- Multiple retractors can be utilized to accomplish a multilevel fusion. However, for fusions extending three or more levels, an alternative retractor system is recommended.

- Design characteristics
  - The addition of an expandable mechanism (or skirt) can enlarge the deepest part of the retractor from 2.4 to 8 cm.
  - These retractors enable the simultaneous visualization of adjacent level pedicles for direct placement of screws and rods.
  - Some retractors have the capability to pivot the proximal aspect of the cylinder thereby increasing visualization at the base of the wound.
- Design limitations
  - The static narrow proximal aperture requires the utilization of specialized instrumentation and limits the angulation potential despite the enlarged deepest part of the retractor. This may create a steep learning curve for surgeons.
  - To adequately expand the retractor at the base of the wound, a significant amount soft tissue may need to be dissected.

Expandable Blade Retractors (Fig. 2.8)

- Design purpose
  - Independently expandable retractor blades provide a larger exposure of the surgical field and allow the utilization of instruments and technical skills utilized in traditional open surgery (minimizing the steep learning curve).
  - These retractors have inherent flexibility to adjust to variations in the local anatomy.
- Design characteristics
  - Three to four separate retractor blades can expand independently in a cranial-caudal and medial-lateral direction to create a surgical corridor.
  - The surgical corridor is larger and can adapt to maximize exposure for up to two levels.

Pitfalls

- The tubular and blade retractor systems require attachment to a table mounted rigid or flexible arm. If the patient's position shifts during the procedure, the surgical field can become compromised.
- Minimal expansion of the retractor limits tissue disruption and creep while maintaining adequate visualization.

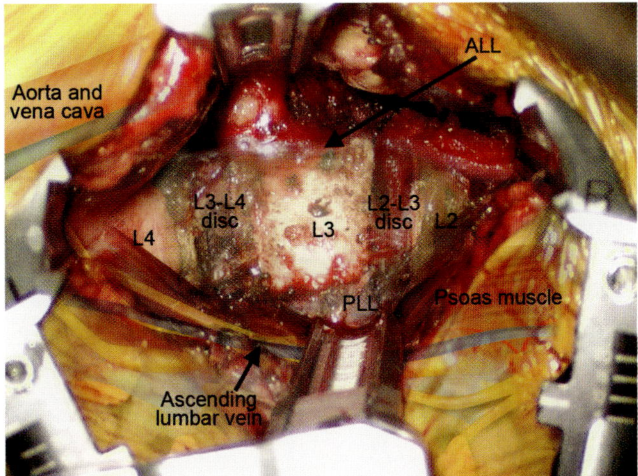

Fig. 2.8: Four blade expandable retractors are utilized to increase the visualization of the operative field during a lateral lumbar corpectomy.

  - The blades are assembled individually onto a fixed frame containing glide rails that allow independent microadjustments of the retractor position.
  - To minimize the skin incision, the frame can have a built-in curve or a pivot-point design that promotes greater distal expansion relative to the proximal excursion.
  - Some retractors come with a telescoping extension that can be adjusted to the necessary depth and avoid soft tissue or muscle "creep" into the field.
  - Special design features
    - Some frames allow the intermittent release of tension, which reduces soft tissue pressure during longer operations.
    - During an interbody fusion through an extreme lateral approach, a retractor with a built-in neuromonitoring capability can help protect the nerve structures during the procedure. Repositioning of the retractor is done as necessary to avoid neural injury.
- Design limitations
  - The greater exposure and visualization of the surgical wound comes at the expense of greater soft tissue dissection and tension, which may be accompanied by greater postoperative pain.
  - The retractor system requires a relatively complicated assembly process that can add to the intraoperative time.
  - The retractor blade design can result in tissue creep obstructing visualization of the surgical field.

Pedicle Screw-based Retractors—Thoracic and Lumbar Spine (Fig. 2.9)

- Design purpose
  - The pedicle screw-based retractor system is attached to the spine itself, stabilizing the surgical field irrespective of the patient's position on the operating table.
  - This retractor system also significantly decreases the setup time associated with conventional table-mounted retractor systems.
- Design characteristics
  - Under fluoroscopic guidance the pedicle screws attached to the flexible retractor sleeve are introduced percutaneously.
    - A cannulated access needle is inserted through the pedicle to the desired depth within the vertebral body.
    - A guidewire is then placed through the cannula, and the access needle is removed. An incision is then made in the skin, and the fascia is incised inline.
    - The pedicle is tapped and the screw with the attached flexible retractor sleeve is inserted. This process is repeated as needed, depending on the number of levels involved.
  - Gelpi retractors are utilized to spread the flexible retractor sleeves and expose the pedicle screw heads.
  - A rod is then introduced from the end screw and passed through each of the screw heads under direct visualization.

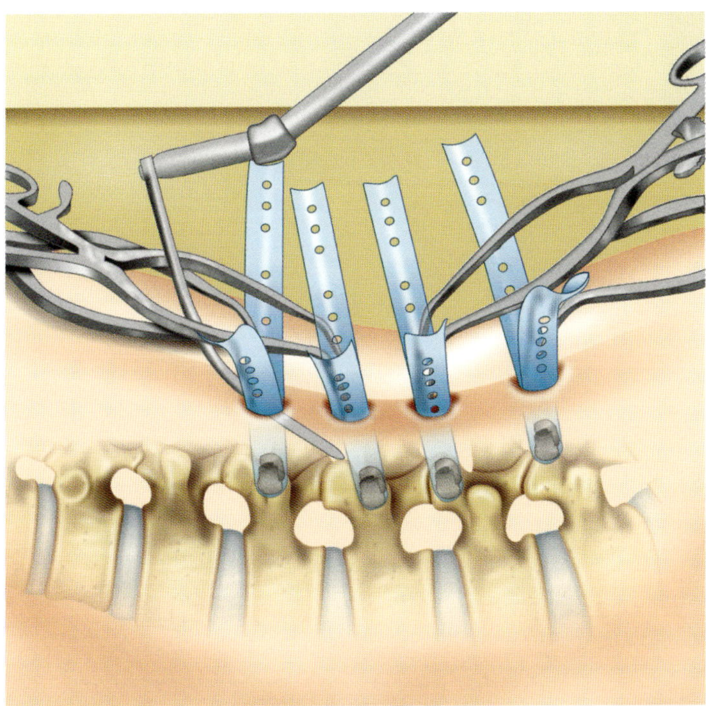

Fig. 2.9: Artist rendering of pedicle screw-based retractor system. Redrawn with permission from Serengeti, K2M, Inc, Leesburg, VA.

    - Special design feature (lumbar interbody fusion).
        - A separate screw-based expandable blade retractor that works in conjunction with the flexible retractor sleeve can be utilized. This combination can achieve simultaneous cranial-caudal, medial-lateral retraction and disc space distraction in one single step.
- Design limitations
    - The flexible sleeve retractors are prone to breakage under undue tension.
    - If the screw is inserted too deep into the vertebral body, removal of the retractor sleeve can be difficult.
    - Despite its advantages, this retractor system is limited to only posterior interbody fusions and instrumentation in the lumbar spine.
    - Undue retraction/pressure may compromise the pedicle screw fixation.

CONCLUSION

- The goals of minimally invasive spine surgery include reduced iatrogenic muscle injury leading to reduced postoperative pain and expedited functional recovery.[1,2]
- Recent advancements in tubular retractor design have expanded the reach of minimally invasive spine surgery to a wide variety of degenerative, traumatic, and neoplastic processes in all areas of the spine. Excellent outcomes combined with fewer complications, shorter hospital stays, and less blood loss have been reported.[3]

- Minimally invasive paramedian incisions and self-retaining retractors have eliminated the need for aggressive soft tissue disruption and tendon detachment associated with open procedures while still achieving the goals of the surgery. This leads to improved postoperative dynamic stability of the spine.[2]

REFERENCES

1. Celestre PC, Pazmino PR, Mikhael MM, et al. Minimally invasive approaches to the cervical spine. Orthop Clin North Am. 2012;43:137-47, x.
2. Kim CW. Scientific basis of minimally invasive spine surgery—prevention of multifidus muscle injury during posterior lumbar surgery. Spine 2010;35: S281-6.
3. Kazemi N CL, Tredway TL. The future of spine surgery—new horizons in the treatment of spinal disorders. Surg Neurol Int. 2013;4(Suppl 1):S15-21.

REFERENCE SUMMARY

1. Celestre PC, Pazmino PR, Mikhael MM, et al. Minimally invasive approaches to the cervical spine. The Orthopedic Clinics of North America 2012;43:137-47.
   Summary: A literature review describing the goals, indications, contraindications, surgical techniques, and positive outcomes associated with minimally invasive cervical spine surgery. The authors conclude that a minimally invasive approach to the cervical spine is associated with improved postoperative pain, decreased blood loss, and equivalent clinical outcomes when compared with an open approach.
2. Kim CW. Scientific Basis of Minimally Invasive Spine Surgery—prevention of multifidus muscle injury during posterior lumbar surgery. Spine 2010;35: S281-6.
   Summary: A literature review regarding the scientific and anatomic basis of minimally invasive spine surgery. The authors describe how a minimally invasive posterior approach to the lumbar spine avoids injury to the musculotendinous complex and the neurovascular bundles.
3. Kazemi N CL, Tredway TL. The future of spine surgery—New horizons in the treatment of spinal disorders. Surgical Neurology International 2013;4(Supple 1): S15-S21.
   Summary: A literature review describing the advancements in spine surgery with regards to minimally invasive approaches, robotics and navigation, motion preservation, and biologics. The authors report that due to the recent improvements of retractor systems, a wide variety of pathologies can be treated via a minimally invasive approach with excellent outcomes, fewer complications, shorter hospital stays, and less blood loss than conventional open procedures.

Chapter 3

Minimally Invasive Posterior Cervical Foraminotomy

Alejandro Marquez-Lara, Alpesh A Patel, Kern Singh

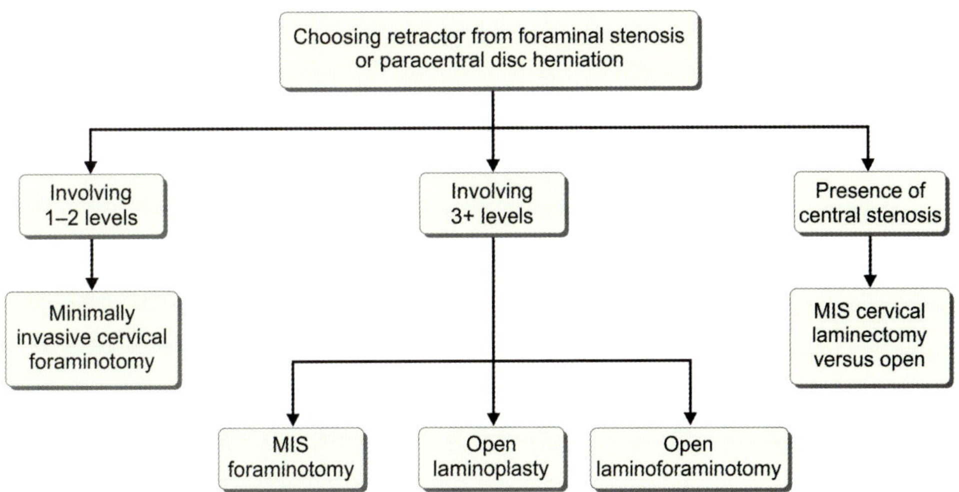

CASE VIGNETTE

A 57-year-old woman presents to the office with a 6-month history of pain, numbness, and tingling in her left upper extremity. The pain begins in her neck and shoulder and radiates into her radial two digits. On examination, the patient has left sided C6 radicular symptoms with motor weakness noticeable with wrist extension on the left side. There are no signs or symptoms of myelopathy. The patient's symptoms are refractory to conservative management with physical therapy and analgesic medication.

DIAGNOSTIC IMAGING

- Plain film radiography—Anteroposterior and lateral views (flexion-extension)
  - Important to rule out instability that may necessitate a cervical fusion
- Magnetic resonance imaging (MRI) (Fig. 3.1)
  - Necessary to evaluate the etiology and severity of the neural compression

Imaging Pearls

- Parasagittal and oblique MRI images (T1 weighted) can help determine the severity of foraminal stenosis.
- CT myelography is the preferred imaging modality for the evaluation of spinal cord compression secondary to bone and in patients with previously placed instrumentation.

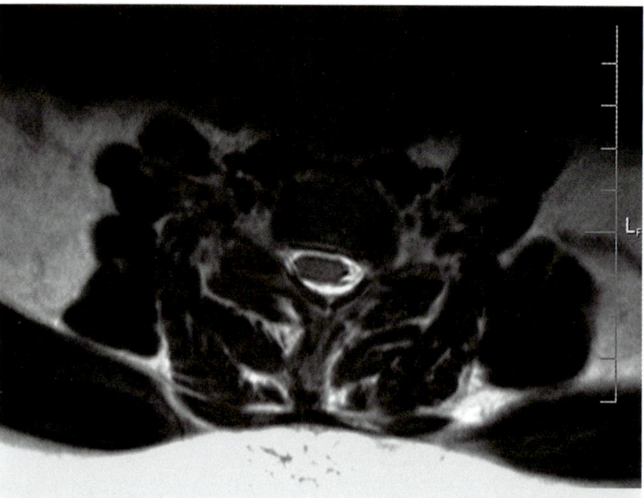

Fig. 3.1: Preoperative axial magnetic resonance image demonstrating left foraminal stenosis at C4–C5 with minimal central stenosis.

- Computed tomography (CT)
  - Helpful in determining soft disc herniation from bony osteophyte or calcified disc herniation
  - CT myelography is useful in patients who are unable to undergo an MRI (ocular implants, cardiac pacemaker).

SURGICAL INDICATIONS

- Single or multilevel paracentral/foraminal herniated nucleus pulposus (HNP)
- Isolated spondylotic foraminal stenosis
- Multilevel spondylotic foraminal stenosis without central stenosis
- Persistent radicular symptoms after anterior cervical discectomy and fusion or anterior cervical disc replacement
- Contraindications to an anterior approach
  - Superficial infection
  - Tracheostomy
  - History of anterior neck radiation

Indication Pearls

- HNP location in regards to the spinal cord (central) and nerve root (foramen) will help determine if the disc can be accessed posteriorly.

Contraindications

- Central disc herniation or osteophytes
- Myelopathy from central canal stenosis
- Ossification of posterior longitudinal ligament (OPLL)
- Kyphotic deformity
- Cervical segment instability

INSTRUMENTATION

- Intraoperative fluoroscopy
- Microscope
- Sequential dilators
- Tubular retractor (16–21 mm) with mounted retractor arm
- Microscopic instruments
  - Rongeurs
    - Pituitary
    - Kerrison
  - Microcurettes
  - High-speed burr

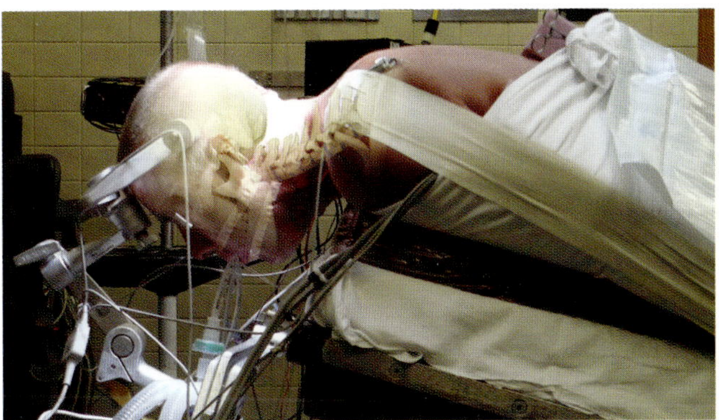

Fig. 3.2: The patient is placed in a prone position with the neck gently flexed to open the spinal canal.

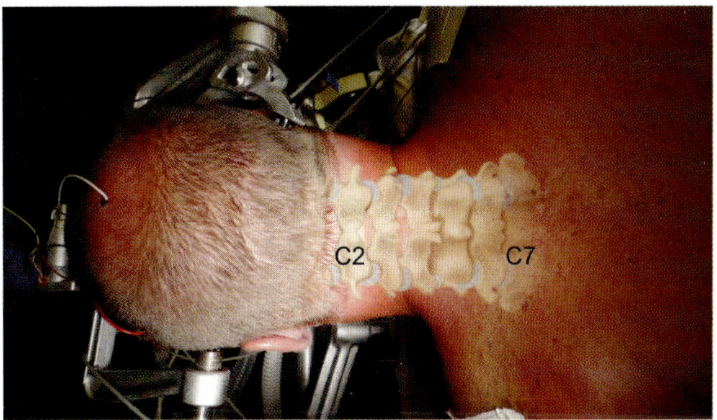

Fig. 3.3: Topographic anatomy of the posterior cervical spine highlighting the C2 and C7 spinous processes that can be palpated to identify the precise surgical site.

POSITIONING AND INTRAOPERATIVE SETUP

- Endotracheal intubation is performed in a supine position.
- The patient is fitted into a Mayfield three-point fixation holder or into Gardner-Wells tongs.
- Modified prone position
  - The patient is placed into a prone position.
    - Appropriate padding is placed over bony prominences.
    - Log rolls are placed along the chest to relieve intra-abdominal pressure. Alternatively, an open frame Jackson table can be utilized.
  - The bed is adjusted to bring the patient into a 30° reverse Trendelenburg position. This elevates the surgical site above the heart to reduce venous bleeding.
  - The head is slightly forward flexed opening the spinal canal (Fig. 3.2).
- Semi-sitting position
  - From a supine position, patient is flexed into a sitting position such that the long axis of the cervical spine is perpendicular to the floor.
- The surgeon is positioned on the ipsilateral side of the surgical site.
- Fluoroscopy and image monitors are placed on the contralateral side of the surgical site.

Positioning Pearls

- Flex the patient's knees prior to changing the bed position to prevent the patient from sliding downward.
- Taping the shoulders down will help expose the lower cervical levels during intraoperative imaging.

Positioning Pitfalls

- There is a risk of air emboli with a semi-sitting position. A precordial Doppler may be utilized to monitor for this rare adverse event.

Surgical Anatomy and Exposure

- The spinous processes of C2 and C7 can serve as superficial landmarks (Fig. 3.3).
- Lateral fluoroscopic images will help determine the proper surgical level.
- The surgical site is marked and infiltrated with a local anesthetic.
- A longitudinal 15-mm incision is made 5–10 mm lateral to the midline on the ipsilateral side of the pathology.
- A longitudinal fasciotomy is made, equal in length to the skin incision, and the starting dilator is advanced gently under fluoroscopic guidance (Fig. 3.4).

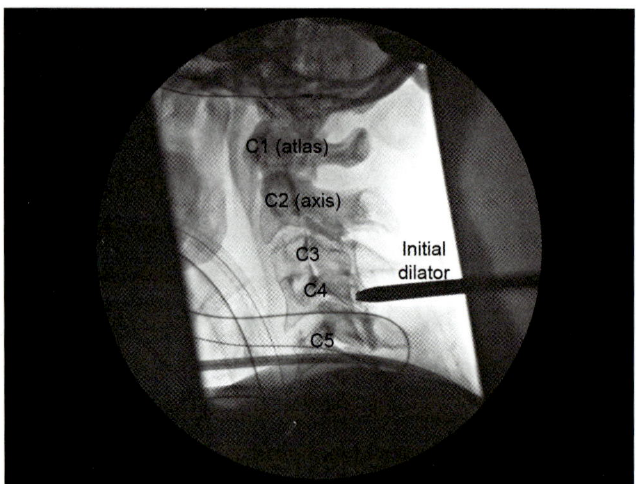

Fig. 3.4: Placement of the initial dilator under lateral fluoroscopic guidance.

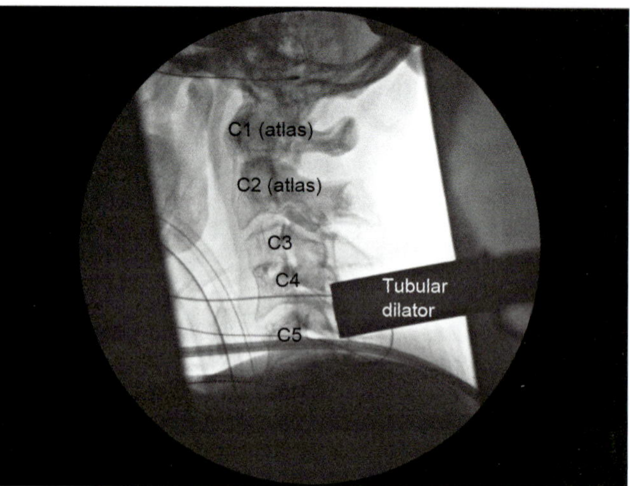

Fig. 3.5: Sequential dilation creates an intermuscular working channel that minimizes soft tissue damage. The final dilator is visualized in the correct position.

- Sequential dilation is performed (Fig. 3.5). Once the final dilator is reached a tubular retractor is placed and locked into the mounted retractor arm.
- Electrocautery and a pituitary rongeur can clear any remaining muscle and soft tissue, exposing the lateral mass, facet joints, and interlaminar space (Fig. 3.6).
  - At this point, a fluoroscopic image is obtained to confirm that the retractor is at the correct level.

PROCEDURE SPECIFIC STEPS

- Step 1
  - With a high-speed burr, the medial third of the inferior articular process of the cephalad vertebra is removed until the superior articular process (SAP) of the caudad vertebra is visualized (Fig. 3.7).
    - A small laminotomy in the superior vertebra may help expose the lateral aspect of the ligamentum flavum overlying the SAP.
    - The ligamentum flavum is carefully excised with a 1- or 2-mm Kerrison rongeur.
- Step 2
  - Next, the medial third of the exposed SAP of the caudal vertebra is resected with a burr or a Kerrison rongeur (Fig. 3.8).
- Step 3
  - With a fine angled dissector, the nerve is inspected from medial to lateral. Palpation ventral to the nerve root is important to identify possible disc fragments or osteophytes.
    - If indicated, the nerve root is retracted superiorly and the herniated disc is removed with a pituitary rongeur.

Anatomy/Exposure Pearls

- A fasciotomy will facilitate sequential dilation.
- If the dilators do not pass smoothly, one can bluntly dissect the fascia and muscles with Metzenbaum scissors.

Anatomy/Exposure Pitfalls

- The K-wire and smaller dilators pose a potential risk to penetrate the interlaminar space and should be avoided.

Step 1 Pearls

- The SAP is the source of bony compression and impingement in the dorsal part of the foramen.

Step 2 Pearls

- Palpating the size of the facet with a bayoneted Penfield no. 4 lateral to the tubular retractor can help assess the extent of resection without having to expose the entire facet capsule.
- The laminar-facet junction can be utilized as a landmark to determine the limit of facet resection.

Step 2 Pitfalls

- During resection, the epineural venous plexus may be encountered. Hemostasis can be obtained with a bipolar cautery, bone wax, or a thrombotic agent.
- Removing >50% of the facet joint complex can lead to postoperative neck pain and spinal instability.

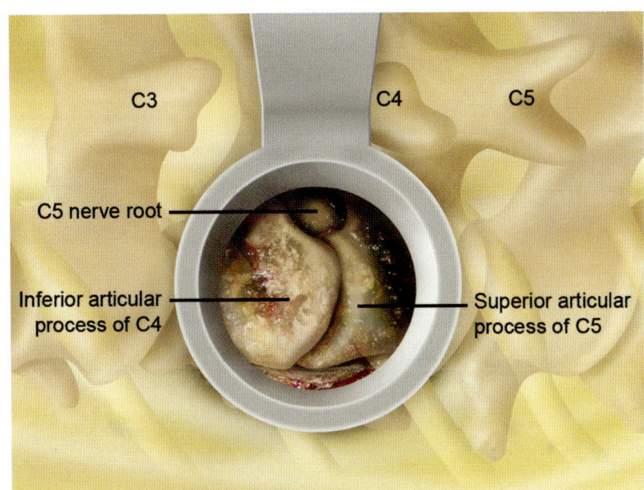

Fig. 3.6: Intraoperative view of the surgical channel after removing the residual soft tissue. The superior and inferior articular processes are clearly identified.

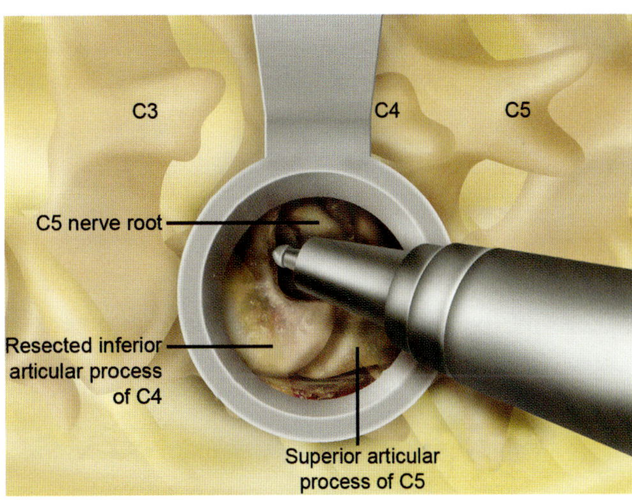

Fig. 3.7: A high-speed burr is displayed removing the medial third of the inferior articular process.

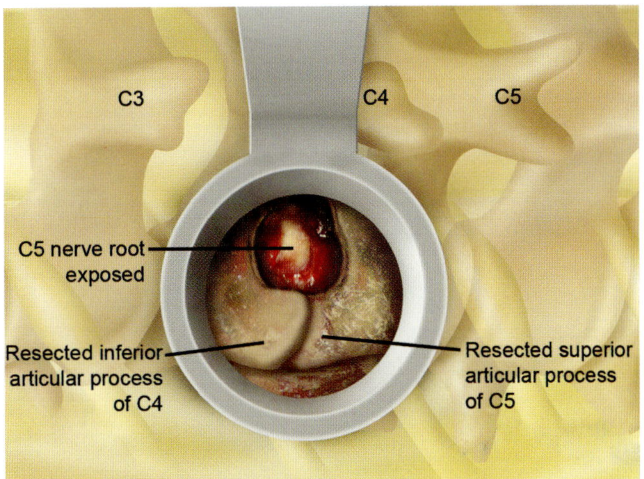

Fig. 3.8: An intraoperative view of the exposed nerve root after partial resection of the inferior and superior articular processes.

- Step 4
    - A final assessment is performed above, below, and medial to the nerve root. Decompression is complete when a nerve probe can be easily passed into the neuroforamen.
- Step 5
    - Copious irrigation of the wound with antibiotic solution and adequate hemostasis is assured prior to wound closure.
    - Final infiltration of local anesthetic to the surgical site will alleviate postoperative pain.
    - Multilayer closure should be performed given the risk of infection with posterior cervical procedures.

Step 3 Pearls

- Additional drilling of the superomedial quadrant of the caudal pedicle improves access to clear ventral debris or disc material and avoids excessive retraction of the nerve root.

Step 3 Pitfalls

- Care must be taken to prevent injury to the anterior motor branch, which can be mistaken for disc material.

POSTOPERATIVE CARE

Complications

- Superficial wound infections
  - Most resolve with oral antibiotics.
  - If necessary, the wound can be formally irrigated and debrided.
- Incidental durotomy
  - Intraoperatively, the durotomy can be covered with muscle, fat, or gel foam followed by a fibrin glue or synthetic sealant.
  - For larger durotomies, a lumbar cerebrospinal fluid (CSF) diverting drain may be placed for 2 to 3 days to prevent a wound leak.
  - Risk of a postoperative pseudomeningocele and CSF-cutaneous fistula are exceedingly rare due to the minimal dead space around the surgical site.
- Transient nerve root paresis
  - Occur from post-manipulation edema and concurrent revascularization of the ischemic nerve root
  - The C5 nerve root is the most frequently involved.
  - Presents 24–48 hours after surgery
  - Close observation and reimaging is indicated to assess for any residual compressive pathology.
  - Most resolve with conservative management.

Complication Pearls

- The C5 nerve root has the most horizontal trajectory and the sharpest angle between the nerve root and the lateral margin of the dura.

EXPECTED AND ADVERSE OUTCOMES

- Minimally invasive posterior cervical foraminotomy provides symptomatic relief in 87–97% of patients with radicular symptoms from foraminal stenosis or a paracentral herniated intervertebral disc.[1-4]
- Intraoperative blood loss, hospital length of stay, and the need for postoperative analgesics are significantly reduced with a minimally invasive approach.[1-4]
- Expected complication rate after a minimally invasive posterior cervical foraminotomy ranges from 2–9%.
  - CSF leak, superficial wound infections and nerve root paresis are the most common postoperative complications.

REFERENCES

1. Hilton DL Jr. Minimally invasive tubular access for posterior cervical foraminotomy with three-dimensional microscopic visualization and localization with anterior/posterior imaging. Spine J: Official Journal of the North American Spine Society. 2007;7:154-8.
2. Winder MJ, Thomas KC. Minimally invasive versus open approach for cervical laminoforaminotomy. Can J Neurol Sci. 2011;38:262-7.
3. Caglar YS, Bozkurt M, Kahilogullari G, et al. Keyhole approach for posterior cervical discectomy: experience on 84 patients. Minimally invasive neurosurgery: MIN. 2007;50:7-11.
4. Witzmann A, Hejazi N, Krasznai L. Posterior cervical foraminotomy. A follow-up study of 67 surgically treated patients with compressive radiculopathy. Neurosurg Rev 2000;23:213-7.

REFERENCE SUMMARY

1. Hilton DL Jr. The authors analyzed the outcomes of a minimally invasive posterior cervical foraminotomy with a standard operating microscope. The surgical outcomes of 222 patients after an average follow-up of 2 years demonstrated symptom improvement in 210 patients (94.6%), improved pain in 9 patients (4.1%), and persistent or worsening pain in 3 patients (1.3%).
2. Winder et al. The authors conducted a retrospective case-control study of 107 patients who underwent a posterior cervical foraminotomy [open vs microscopic tubular assisted foraminotomy (MTPF)]. The MTPF approach demonstrated similar results compared with an open approach while significantly reducing blood loss, postoperative analgesic requirements, and the length of hospital stay.
3. Caglar et al. The authors report on 84 patients who underwent a posterior keyhole laminotomy-foraminotomy under a surgical microscope and discuss the surgical technique, advantages, and disadvantages. This study demonstrated that in select patients, a "keyhole approach" provides excellent results with minimal morbidity.
4. Witzmann et al. A retrospective review of 67 patients with unilateral intraforaminal disease who underwent a posterior cervical foraminotomy under microscope visualization. After an average of 3-year follow-up, 93% of patients experienced complete or partial relief of symptoms. The authors conclude that careful patient selection and microsurgical techniques are essential for obtaining consistent results.

Chapter 4

Minimally Invasive Posterior Cervical Laminectomy and Fusion

Sreeharsha V Nandyala, Damandeep Singh Makkar, Alpesh A Patel

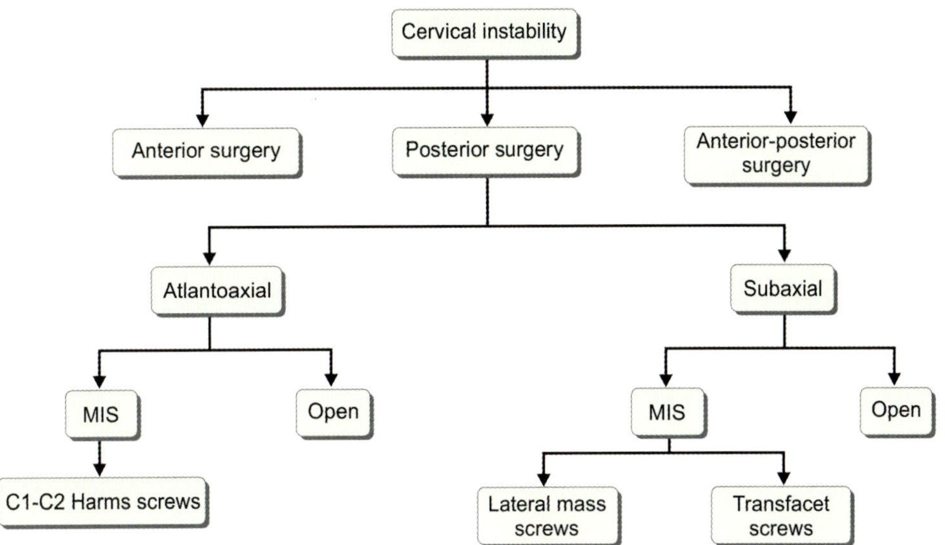

C1–C2 FUSION

Case Vignette

A 47-year-old woman with a history of rheumatoid arthritis (RA) presents to the office with neck pain that radiates to the occiput and worsens with forward flexion. In addition, the patient reports worsening gait and a loss of fine motor dexterity of the upper extremities. She denies any recent trauma. Physical examination demonstrates bilateral positive Hoffman's sign, generalized lower extremity hyper-reflexia, diminished position sense in the toes, and gait imbalance.

Diagnostic Imaging

- Plain film radiography (Figs. 4.1A and B)
  - Anteroposterior (AP) and lateral views (flexion-extension)
  - Open mouth (ADI and lateral mass displacement)

C1–C2 Imaging Pearls

- Radiographic signs of significant instability: (1) atlanto dens interval (ADI) >3 mm; (2) Spinal canal diameter <13 mm (3) posterior atlanto dens interval (PADI) <12 mm.
- The size of the vertebra will guide the decision to safely place C2 fixation (a transarticular screw, C2 pedicle or pars screw, or C2 laminar screw).

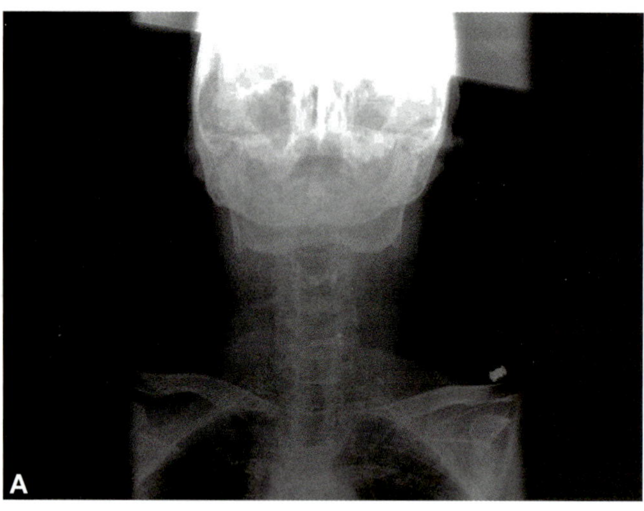

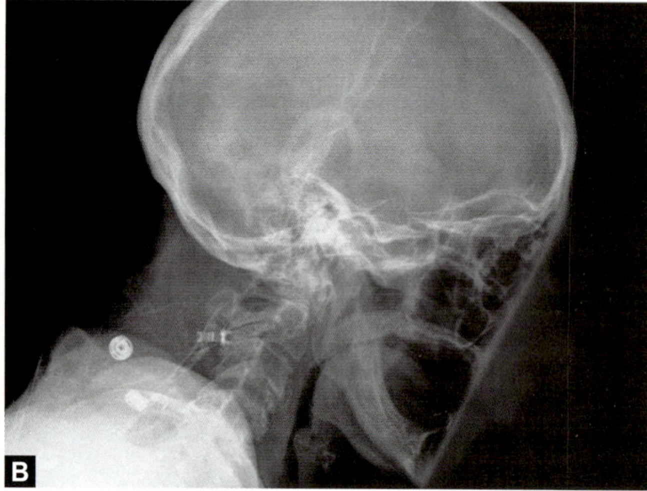

Figs. 4.1A and B: Preoperative (A) anteroposterior and (B) lateral radiograph demonstrating C1–C2 spondylosis.

- Computed tomography (CT)
  - Axial and sagittal reconstruction provides detail of the bony anatomy, including the foramen transversarium and vertebral artery.
- Magnetic resonance imaging (MRI)
  - May help assess the integrity of the transverse ligament of the atlas
  - Will identify concurrent conditions in RA (C1-2 pannus with cord compression, basilar invagination with brainstem compression, subaxial subluxations)

Surgical Indications

- Atlantoaxial instability
  - Traumatic
    - Rupture of the transverse ligament of the atlas
    - Comminuted type II and III odontoid fractures
    - Adjacent fracture of C1 and C2
    - Rotatory subluxation
  - Congenital
    - Odontoid hypoplasia
    - Os odontoideum
    - Occipitalization of C1 with C1-C2 instability
    - Congenital malformation (i.e. Klippel-Feil syndrome)
  - Inflammatory
    - RA
    - Ankylosis spondylitis
  - C1-C2 osteoarthritis
  - Iatrogenic
    - Nonunions
      - Failed posterior C1-C2 fusion
  - Infectious
    - Osteomyelitis
  - Tumors

Controversies

- In traumatic settings, a more traditional approach may be utilized because of the distorted anatomy. Image guidance can help significantly if a percutaneous stabilization is performed.

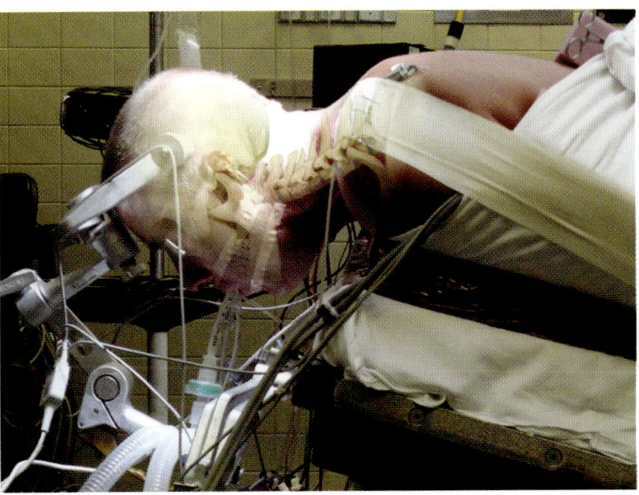

Fig. 4.2: Patient is placed prone on the operating room table with a Mayfield head holder gently flexing the neck.

Instrumentation

- Intraoperative fluoroscopy or advanced image guidance
- Jackson table
- Mayfield head positioner/tongs
- Microscope or magnifying loops
- Retractor
  - Tubular retractors (16–21 mm)
- Rongeurs
  - Pituitary
  - Kerrison
- Microcurettes and angled curettes
- High-speed burr
- Guidewires (Kirschner)
- Screws
  - C1 lateral mass and C2 pars

Positioning and Intraoperative Setup

- Endotracheal intubation is performed in a supine position.
- Neurophysiologic monitoring with electromyography and both transcranial motor and somatosensory evoked potentials should be utilized.
- The patient is fitted into a Mayfield three-point fixation holder.
- Patient position
  - The patient is placed into a prone position (Fig. 4.2).
    - Appropriate padding is placed over the bony prominences.
    - Log rolls are positioned along the chest to relieve intra-abdominal pressure.
      - Alternatively, an open frame Jackson table can be utilized.
  - If necessary, the C1–C2 joint is reduced with gentle extension and traction while applying mild rotation to the chin caudally.

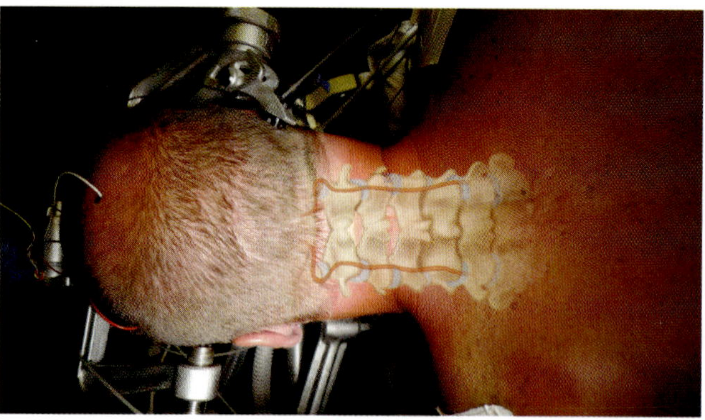

Fig. 4.3: Topographic bony anatomy depicting the trajectory of the vertebral artery in the cervical spine.

  - Tuck the chin to minimize overlap of the occiput with the dorsal arch of C1.
  - The bed is adjusted to bring the patient into a 30° reverse Trendelenburg position. This elevates the surgical site above the heart to reduce venous bleeding.
- Fluoroscopy monitors are placed on the contralateral side of the surgeon.

SURGICAL ANATOMY

Neurovascular Structures

- Carotid artery
  - The internal carotid artery is 2–4 mm from the anterior cortex of the C1 lateral mass in the neutral position.
- Vertebral artery
  - At the C1 level, the vertebral artery traverses cranially 1.5 cm from the midline (Fig. 4.3).
- First and second cervical spinal nerves
  - The C1 nerve root lies in the groove of the posterior arch along with the vertebral artery, posterior to the lateral mass of the atlas.
  - The C2 nerve root lies dorsal to the C1–C2 articulation between the posterior arches.
    - Large epidural venous sinuses are located around the C2 nerve, so bleeding may be common.

Anatomy Pearls

- In 3–15% of patients, the vertebral artery is contained within the arcuate foramen. The arcuate foramen is formed by a thin bony arch (ponticulus posticus). Care must be taken to identify this structure as it can be mistaken for the C1 lamina. Preoperative CT imaging is helpful.

PROCEDURE-SPECIFIC STEPS

C1 Lateral Mass and C2 Pars Screw-rod Construct—Harms Technique (Figs. 4.4A to D)

- Step 1
  - Under fluoroscopic guidance, a spinal needle is inserted 5–10 mm lateral to the midline in a trajectory parallel to the C2 spinous process.

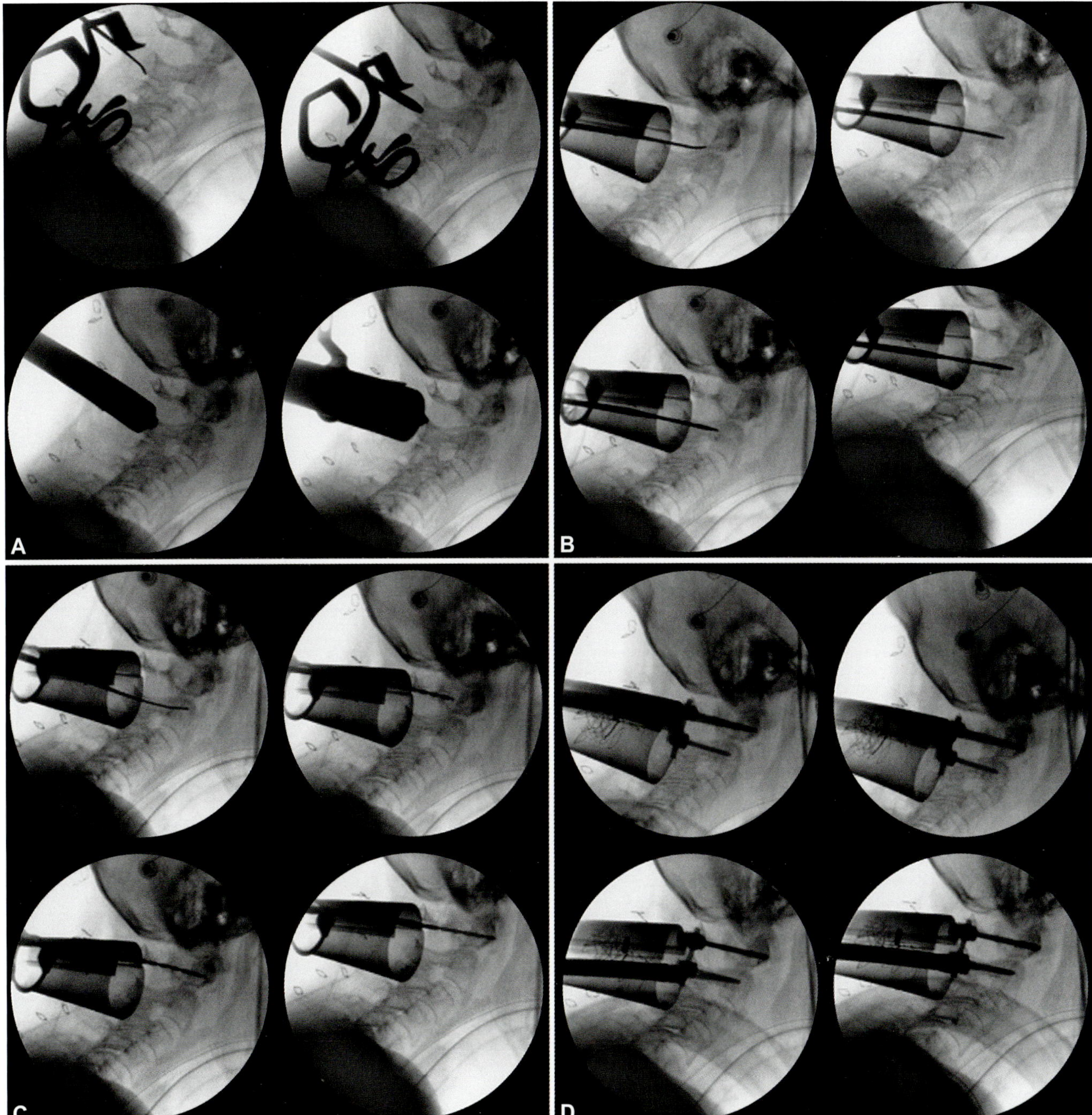

Figs. 4.4A to D: C1–C2 fixation as described in the report by Taghva et al.[12]

- The spinal needle is then advanced until it reaches the C2 lateral mass.
- A 20–30 mm longitudinal skin incision is performed centered on the entry point of the spinal needle.
- A longitudinal fasciotomy is performed, equal in length to the skin incision, and the starting dilator is advanced gently under fluoroscopic guidance.

- Step 2
  - Sequential dilation is performed through an intermuscular paraspinal plane.
  - The trajectory of the tube should be directed laterally to dock on the C1–C2 facet.
  - Once the final dilator is reached, an expandable retractor is placed and locked into the mounted retractor arm.
  - Electrocautery and a pituitary rongeur may be used to clear any remaining muscle and soft tissue to expose the lateral mass and facet joints.
    - The surface anatomy of the lamina, facet, and lateral masses should be clearly identified if the tube placement is correct.
- Step 3
  - The caudal portion of the C1 lateral mass is exposed and bipolar electrocautery of the venous plexus is applied for hemostasis and visualization.
  - Hemostatic agents (gelfoam, thrombin) can be utilized to control bleeding.
  - Subperiosteal dissection of the inferior C1 arch as well as the C1 lateral mass will minimize bleeding.
- Step 4
  - A pilot hole is then drilled at the midpoint of the C1 lateral mass just below the arch.
- Step 5
  - Under lateral fluoroscopy, the C1 screw is oriented in a 10° medial and 20° cephalad direction for bicortical bone purchase.
  - The trajectory of the C1 screw should aim for the inferior to middle 1/3 of the anterior C1 ring on lateral fluoroscopy, otherwise penetration of the O-C1 joint is likely.
  - The C1 screw should not extend to or beyond the anterior surface of the C1 ring, otherwise penetration of the anterior cortex of C1 will occur and place the internal carotid artery at risk.
- Step 6 (Fig. 4.5)[2]
  - The entry point of the C2 pars screw starts in the cephalad and medial quadrant of the C2 isthmus.
  - A pilot hole is made with a 2-mm drill bit to reach the opposite cortex.
    - The trajectory of the drill bit should be at a 20–30° cephalad and medial orientation respecting the medial and superior walls of the C2 isthmus.
    - Direct palpation of the superior and medial surface of the C2 pedicle provides a landmark for assessing screw trajectory.
- Step 7 (Fig. 4.6)
  - After assuring the integrity of the pilot hole with a blunt probe, a 3.5-mm polyaxial bicortical screw of the appropriate length is inserted.
- Step 8 (Figs. 4.7A to D)
  - After the placement of the screws, an appropriate sized rod is passed down the tube and fitted into the cephalad screw heads.
  - Slight elevation of the retractor enables the advancement of the rod to the caudal screw heads.

C1–C2 Lateral Mass Screw Pearls

- Bicortical C1 lateral mass screws carry a risk for internal carotid injury with anterior cortical violation.
- This complication can be avoided with 10° of medial orientation.
- If the initial screw trajectory is drilled into the facet joint, a new starting point can be made 1 mm above the previous starting point and a new path can be drilled with slightly more cephalad angulation.

Pitfalls

- This technique carries a steep learning curve because visualization of the pathologic segment is performed at an angle.
- Bleeding may be encountered if dissection is extended past the lateral mass.

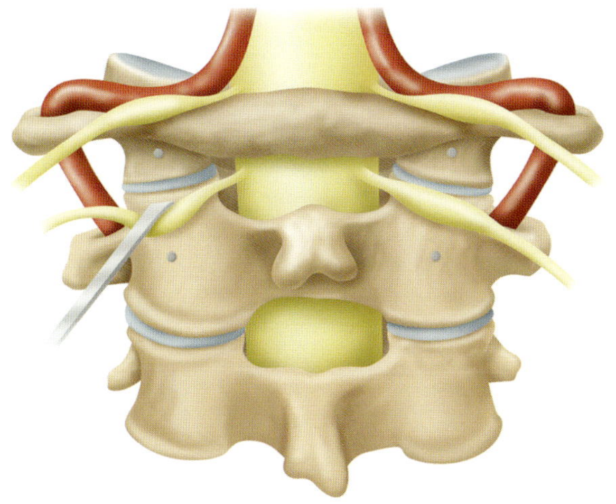

Fig. 4.5: Illustration of a posterior view of the proximal cervical spine demonstrating the entry points at C1 and C2 for screw placement according to the Harm's technique.[2]

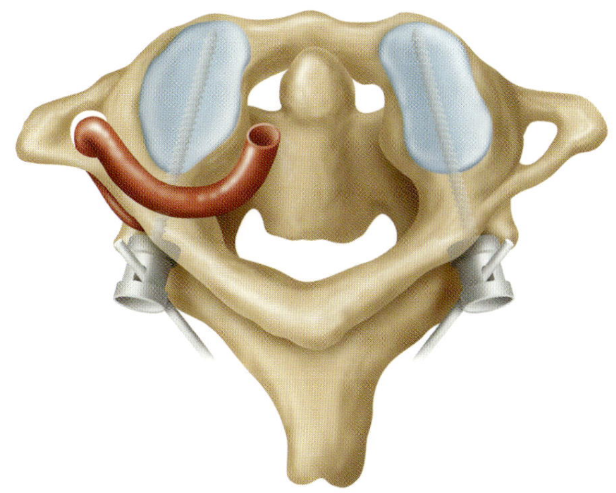

Fig. 4.6: Axial view of the atlas depicting bilateral polyaxial screws placed bicortically into the lateral mass.[2]

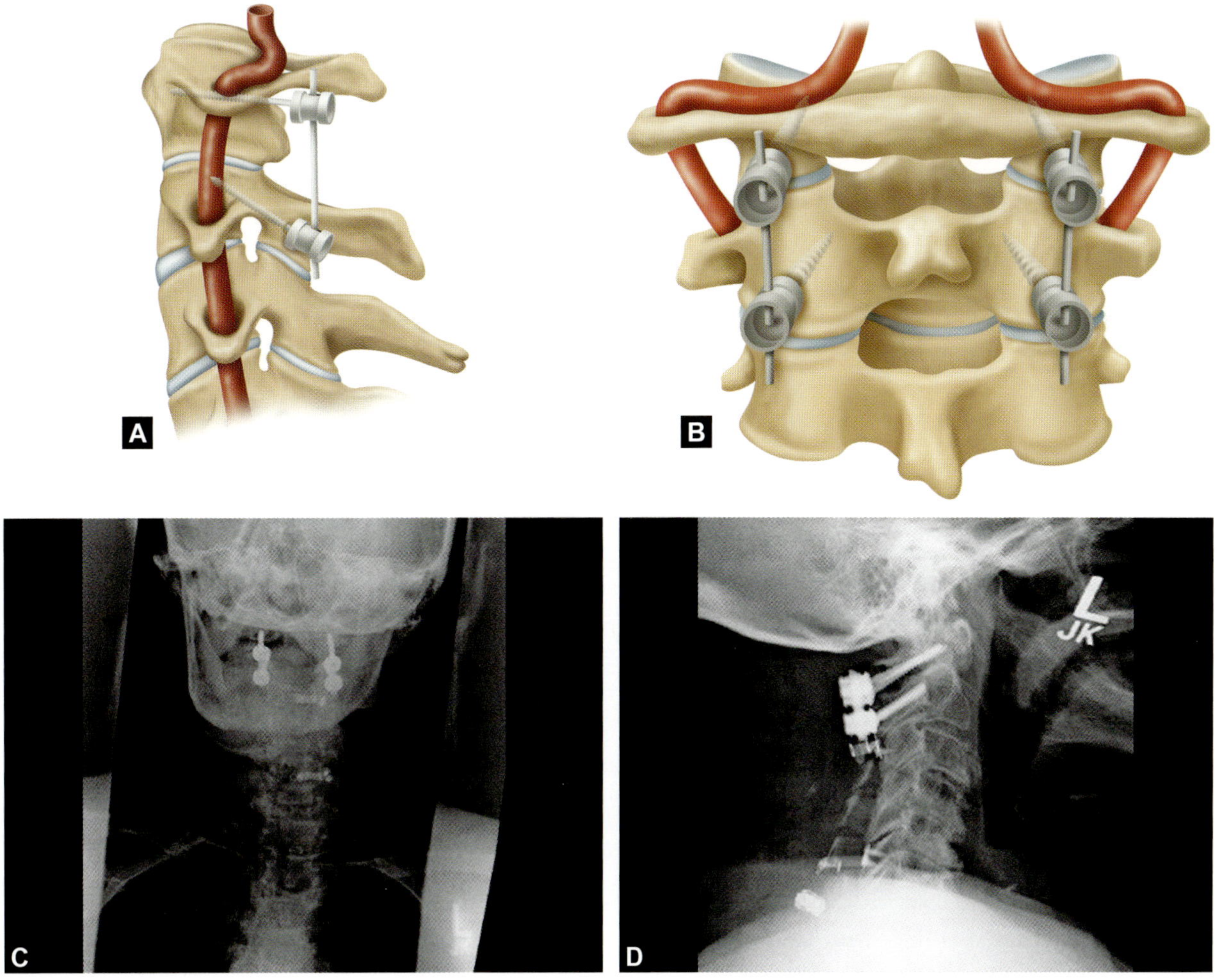

Figs. 4.7A to D: (A and B) Artist representation of final construct after C1–C2 fixation with polyaxial screws. (C and D) Postoperative anteroposterior and lateral radiographs demonstrating well placed C1–C2 screws and rod.[2]

SUBAXIAL LAMINECTOMY AND FUSION

Case Vignette

A 65-year-old man presents to the office with a 9-month history of worsening neck pain and spasms. The patient reports right-sided upper extremity numbness and tingling as well as increasing clumsiness with fine motor activities. On examination, the patient has right-sided C5 radiculopathy and myelopathic hand findings. He demonstrates deltoid motor weakness with arm abduction, a positive Hoffman's sign, and an inverted radial reflex on the right side. There is no evidence of gait ataxia. The patient's symptoms were refractory to conservative management with physical therapy and analgesics.

Diagnostic Imaging

- Plain film radiography (Fig. 4.8)
  - AP and lateral views (flexion-extension)
- CT
  - Axial and sagittal reconstruction provides detail of the bony anatomy, including the foramen transversarium.
- MRI
  - Allows assessment of the cord morphology and the degree of spinal stenosis

Surgical Indications for Cervical Subaxial Laminectomy

- Cervical spondylosis
  - Radiculopathy—Herniated nucleus pulposus (HNP)
  - Myelopathy
- Neoplasm
- Infection with epidural extension
- Ligamentum flavum hypertrophy and calcification

Imaging Pearls

- CT myelography is the preferred imaging modality to evaluate the bony anatomy and neural compression in patients with previously placed instrumentation.

Laminectomy Indication Pearls

- The location of the HNP in relation to the spinal cord (central) will help determine if the disc can be accessed by a posterior approach. In general, the more lateral the HNP, the easier it is to remove via a posterior approach.

Contraindications

- Moderate to severe kyphosis
- Vascular abnormalities
- Predominant neck pain

Laminectomy Controversies

- Patients with a slight loss of cervical lordosis or with a mild kyphosis may be amenable to a minimally invasive posterior laminectomy.

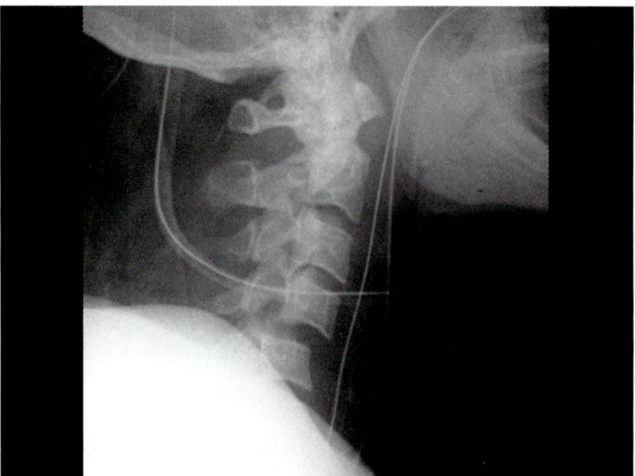

Fig. 4.8: Preoperative lateral radiograph demonstrating C4–C5 bilateral facet dislocation.

SURGICAL INDICATIONS FOR CERVICAL SUBAXIAL FUSION

Subaxial Lateral Mass Screw-rod Construct

- Subaxial instability
  - Traumatic
    - Facet fracture and dislocation
    - Posterior discoligamentous instability
  - Iatrogenic
    - Postlaminectomy syndrome
    - Pseudarthrosis after anterior cervical fusion
  - Infection
  - Tumor

Subaxial Transfacet Screw

- Utilized as an adjunct to anterior cervical fusions

Subaxial Lateral Mass Screws Contraindications

- Anomalous vertebral artery anatomy
- Hypoplastic lateral mass
- Comminuted lateral mass fracture

INSTRUMENTATION

- Intraoperative fluoroscopy or advanced image guidance
- Mayfield head positioner/tongs
- Microscope or magnifying loupes
- Retractor
  - Tubular retractors (16–21 mm) can be utilized for up to two-level fusions.
  - Expandable tubular retractors (20–30 mm) can be utilized for multilevel cases.
- Rongeurs
  - Pituitary
  - Kerrison
- Microcurettes and angled curettes
- High-speed burr
- Guidewire (Kirschner)
- Screws
  - Lateral mass
  - Transfacet

Positioning and Intraoperative Setup

- Endotracheal intubation is performed in a supine position.
- Neurophysiologic monitoring with electromyography and both motor and somatosensory-evoked potentials should be utilized.
- The patient is fitted into a Mayfield three-point fixation holder.
- Modified prone position
  - The patient is placed into a prone position (*see* Fig. 4.2).
    - Appropriate padding is placed over the bony prominences.
    - Log rolls are positioned along the chest to relieve intra-abdominal pressure. Alternatively, an open frame Jackson table can be utilized.

Positioning Pearls

Neck position

- For a **laminectomy**, the head is slightly forward-flexed to open the spinal canal.
- For a **fusion** procedure, the neck is placed in a neutral position to avoid fixation in extension or flexion.

Positioning Pitfalls

- There is a theoretical risk of air embolism with a semi-sitting position. A precordial Doppler should be utilized to monitor for this complication.

  - The bed is adjusted to bring the patient into a 30° reverse Trendelenburg position. This elevates the surgical site above the heart to reduce venous bleeding.
- Semi-sitting position
  - From a supine position, the patient is flexed into a sitting position such that the long axis of the cervical spine is perpendicular to the floor.
- The Mayfield holder is tightened and is subsequently secured to the bed on a U-frame.
- Fluoroscopy monitors are placed on the contralateral side of the surgeon.

Surgical Anatomy

- Subaxial cervical vertebrae
  - Thin laminae
  - Small, medially oriented pedicles
  - Facet joints
    - Composed of the superior and inferior articular processes of the lateral masses.
    - Joint line is coronal in orientation with 45° of cephalad-caudal angulation.
- Vertebral artery (*see* Fig. 4.3)
  - Ascends from the respective subclavian artery anterior to the longus-colli muscles at C7–T1.
  - Enters the spinal column at C6.
  - At the C1 level, the vertebral artery traverses cranially 1.5 cm from the midline.
    - Care must be taken to avoid screw placement beyond 1.5 cm of the midline at the C1–C2 level.

Anatomy Pearls

- In 5% of the population, the vertebral artery will pass through the C7 transverse foramen. As such, avoidance of the foramen transversarium at C7 may be important during instrumentation of the pedicle and lateral mass.[1]

SURGICAL TECHNIQUES

Subaxial Laminectomy

Surgical Exposure

- The surgical level is determined via lateral fluoroscopic images.
- The surgical site is marked and infiltrated with a local anesthetic with epinephrine.
- A 20–25 mm longitudinal skin incision is made that is 10–15 mm lateral to the midline at the level of interest.
- A longitudinal fasciotomy is made equal in length to the skin incision and the starting dilator is advanced gently under fluoroscopic guidance (Fig. 4.9).
- Sequential tube dilation is performed through an intermuscular paraspinal plane (Fig. 4.10).
- Once the final dilator is reached, a tubular retractor is placed and locked into the mounted retractor arm.

Exposure Pearls

- The guidewire and the smaller dilators can penetrate the interlaminar space. Dissection can be performed with a Metzenbaum scissor to prevent iatrogenic perforation of the interlaminar space.

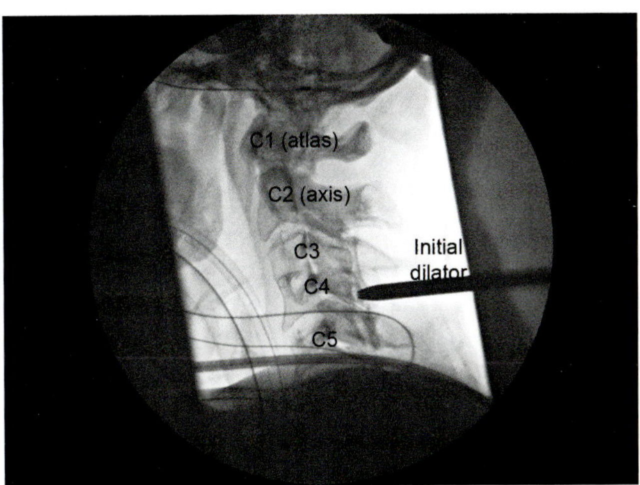

Fig. 4.9: Placement of the initial dilator under lateral fluoroscopic guidance after verification of the correct surgical level.

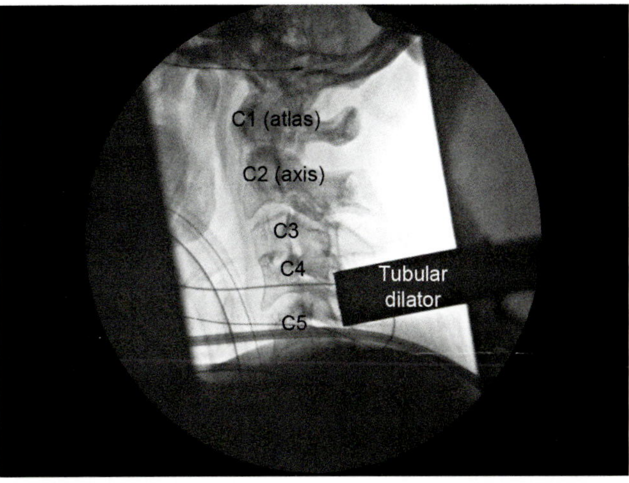

Fig. 4.10: Sequential dilation creates an intermuscular working channel that minimizing soft tissue damage. The final dilator is visualized in the correct position.

- The 16–18-mm tubular retractor should be docked at the lamina-facet junction.
- A medial angulation of the tubular retractor helps in exposing the base of spinous process and the medial edge of the facet joint.

- A long tip electrocautery and a pituitary rongeur can clear any remaining muscle and soft tissue thereby exposing the medial edge of the facet joint.
  - The surface anatomy of the lamina and facet should be clearly identified if the tube placement is correct.

Procedure-specific Steps—Laminectomy

- Step 1
  - An angled curette is utilized to define the cephalad and caudal sublaminar space.
- Step 2
  - A high-speed burr is utilized to remove the inferior part of the superior lamina thereby exposing the attachment of the ligamentum flavum.
  - The laminectomy is continued to the superior part of the inferior lamina.
    - The ligamentum flavum is kept intact whenever possible to protect the dura.
- Step 3
  - The ligamentum flavum is removed with a microscopic curette and Kerrison rongeur.
- Step 4
  - Decompression of the adjacent levels is achieved by angulating the working tube retractor cephalad and caudally.
  - For three or more levels, the incision should be extended and an expandable retractor may be utilized.

Laminectomy Pearls

- During a multilevel laminectomy, the most caudal level should be addressed first to minimize bleeding into the surgical field.
- Approximately 12 mm of bone should be removed to provide an adequate decompression on one side.
- Epidural bleeding can be controlled with the utilization of Cottonoids and thrombogenic agents.
- All adhesions of the ligamentum flavum to the dura should be carefully released with a microcurette.
- Monitor for dural pulsation once the ligamentum flavum is removed.

- Step 5
  - After completing the laminectomy, these same steps are repeated on the contralateral side trough a separate incision.
    - Alternatively, the retractor can be angled medially to decompress the contralateral side. A hooded drill tip should help protect injury to the dura. Care should be taken such that there is no downward pressure applied to the thecal sac and spinal cord.

SUBAXIAL CERVICAL FUSION

Surgical Exposure

- The surgical level is determined via lateral fluoroscopic images.
- The surgical site is marked and infiltrated with a local anesthetic with epinephrine.
- Longitudinal skin incision.
  - Subaxial lateral mass screws: A 20-mm longitudinal midline incision is made.
    - For a single level fusion, the incision should be placed two spinal segments below the level of fusion.
      - This allows the tube trajectory to be parallel to the facet joint at the level of interest.
    - For a multilevel fusion, the incision should be placed one spinal segment above the most caudad level of fusion.
  - Subaxial transfacet screws: A 10–20-mm longitudinal midline incision is made.
    - The incision is generally placed one spinal segment cephalad to the level of interest.
      - If the facet joint has a more horizontal orientation, the incision should be placed more cephalad to accommodate for the screw trajectory.

Exposure Pearls

- For transfacet screws: The more horizontal the plane of the facet joints, the more cephalad the incision.
- Positioning the initial dilators 15–20° cephalad will facilitate instrumentation.

Anatomy/Exposure Pitfalls

- The guidewire and the smaller dilators pose a potential risk to penetrate the interlaminar space.

PROCEDURE-SPECIFIC STEPS—SUBAXIAL LATERAL MASS SCREW-ROD CONSTRUCT

- Step 1
  - A longitudinal fasciotomy is made 5–10 mm lateral to midline that is equal in length to the skin incision. The starting dilator is advanced gently under fluoroscopic guidance.
  - Sequential tube dilation is performed through an intermuscular paraspinal plane.
    - The tube trajectory should be directed laterally to dock on the lateral mass of interest.
    - The tube trajectory should be parallel to the facet joint to facilitate instrumentation.
  - Once the final dilator is reached, a tubular retractor is placed and locked into the mounted retractor arm (Fig. 4.11).
    - For multilevel fixations, it is recommended to use an expandable retractor system (Fig. 4.12).

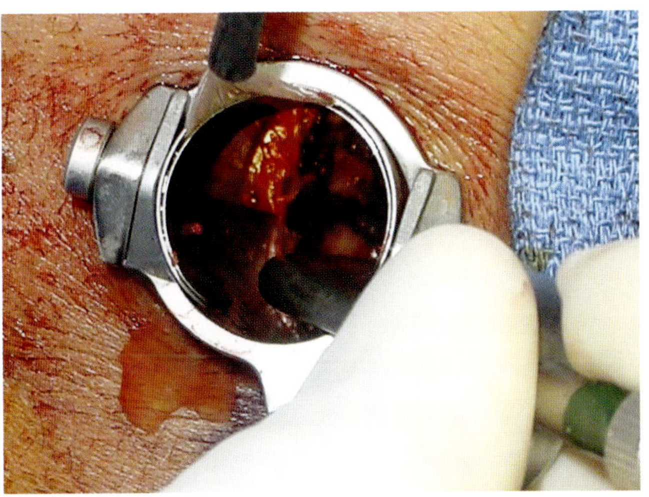

Fig. 4.11: Intraoperative view of a working surgical channel through a tubular retractor.

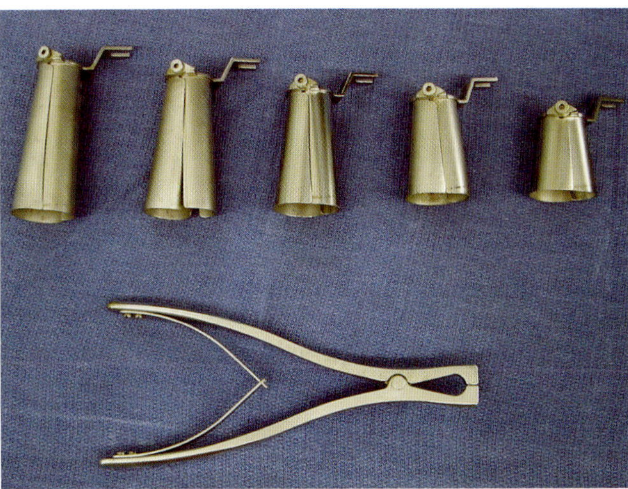

Fig. 4.12: Expandable tubular retractors that are typically utilized for posterior cervical fusion and instrumentation.

  - An electrocautery and a pituitary rongeur can clear any remaining muscle and soft tissue thereby exposing the lateral mass and facet joints.
    - The visualization of both of the facet joints and the medial and lateral edge of the lateral mass will ensure the proper placement of the screws.
    - Visualization will also provide access to the bony surface areas for fusion (lateral mass, facet joints).
- Step 2
  - For the reduction of a locked or perched facet, a burr is utilized to remove part of the superior articular facet from the caudal lateral mass. Subsequent subluxation is achieved as follows:
    - A Penfield instrument is inserted into the joint that is accompanied by a lifting/rotating motion to open the space and allow for reduction.
    - Alternatively, an assistant may use the Mayfield clamp to perform in-line traction and flexion reduction followed by an extension maneuver.
- Step 3
  - The entry point and the trajectory will vary depending upon the technique.[3,4] Once the lateral mass is visualized through the tubular dilator the lateral mass screw technique is very similar to an open procedure. Drilling of the lateral mass screw trajectory is performed under lateral fluoroscopy or image guidance:
    - **An:** The entry point is 1 mm medial to the midpoint of the lateral mass. The direction of the screw is 30° lateral and 15° cephalad (Fig. 4.13A).
    - **Anderson:** The entry point is 1 mm medial to the midpoint of the lateral mass. The direction of the screw is 10° lateral and 30°–45° cephalad (Fig. 4.13B).

Subaxial Lateral Mass Screws Pearls

- Drilling the pilot holes prior to the preparation of the fusion bed and the facet joints is recommended to maintain the anatomic relationships.

Subaxial Lateral Mass Screws Pitfalls

- If the trajectory is too low, it may violate the facet joint and/or the exiting cervical nerve root. If it is too medial it may violate the vertebral artery.

- **Magerl:** Entry point is 1 mm medial and cephalad to the midpoint of the lateral mass. The trajectory of the screw is 25° lateral in the axial plane and parallel to the facet joint in the sagittal plane (30°–45°) (Fig. 4.13C).
  - A prominent spinous process may increase the risk of a lateral screw cutout.
  - This technique enables the placement of a longer screw due to the oblique trajectory.
- **Roy-Camille:** The entry point is at the midpoint of the lateral mass perpendicular to the posterior cortex. The direction of the screw is 10° lateral with no cranial-caudal inclination (Fig. 4.13D).

- Step 4
  - A pilot hole is created with a burr under both direct visualization and lateral fluoroscopic imaging.
  - The drill is then angled according to the methodology above. Once again, the trajectory of the drill is confirmed with adjunct image guidance.
  - If necessary, the pilot hole can be increased in 2 mm increments under fluoroscopic guidance.
- Step 5
  - After all pilot holes are created, the 3.5-mm polyaxial lateral mass screws are inserted through each pilot hole.
- Step 6
  - The fusion bed and facet joints are prepared by decorticating the articular surfaces with a curette.
- Step 7
  - An appropriate sized rod is passed down the tube and manipulated into the cephalad screw heads.
  - Slight elevation of the retractor enables the advancement of the rod to the caudal screw heads.
- At the end of the procedure, the retractor is slowly withdrawn and bipolar cautery is utilized to coagulate vessels behind the retractor.
- The procedure is then repeated through a new paramedian fasciotomy on the contralateral side (Fig. 4.14).

Procedure-Specific Steps—Transfacet Screws[5]

- Step 1
  - A small fascial incision is made overlying the facet involved and a cannulated drill guide is advanced gently under fluoroscopic guidance.
    - The more horizontal the plane of the facet joints, the more cephalad the incision.
  - The drill guide should be docked on the dorsal surface of the superior lateral mass at the level of interest.
- Step 2
  - A pilot hole (14–16 mm) is made at the middle of the superior facet, and a guidewire is advanced until reaching the body of the inferior facet.
    - The trajectory is directed as laterally as possible without fracturing the facet laterally.
    - The caudal orientation should be perpendicular to the facet joint.
      - This may be limited by the occiput.

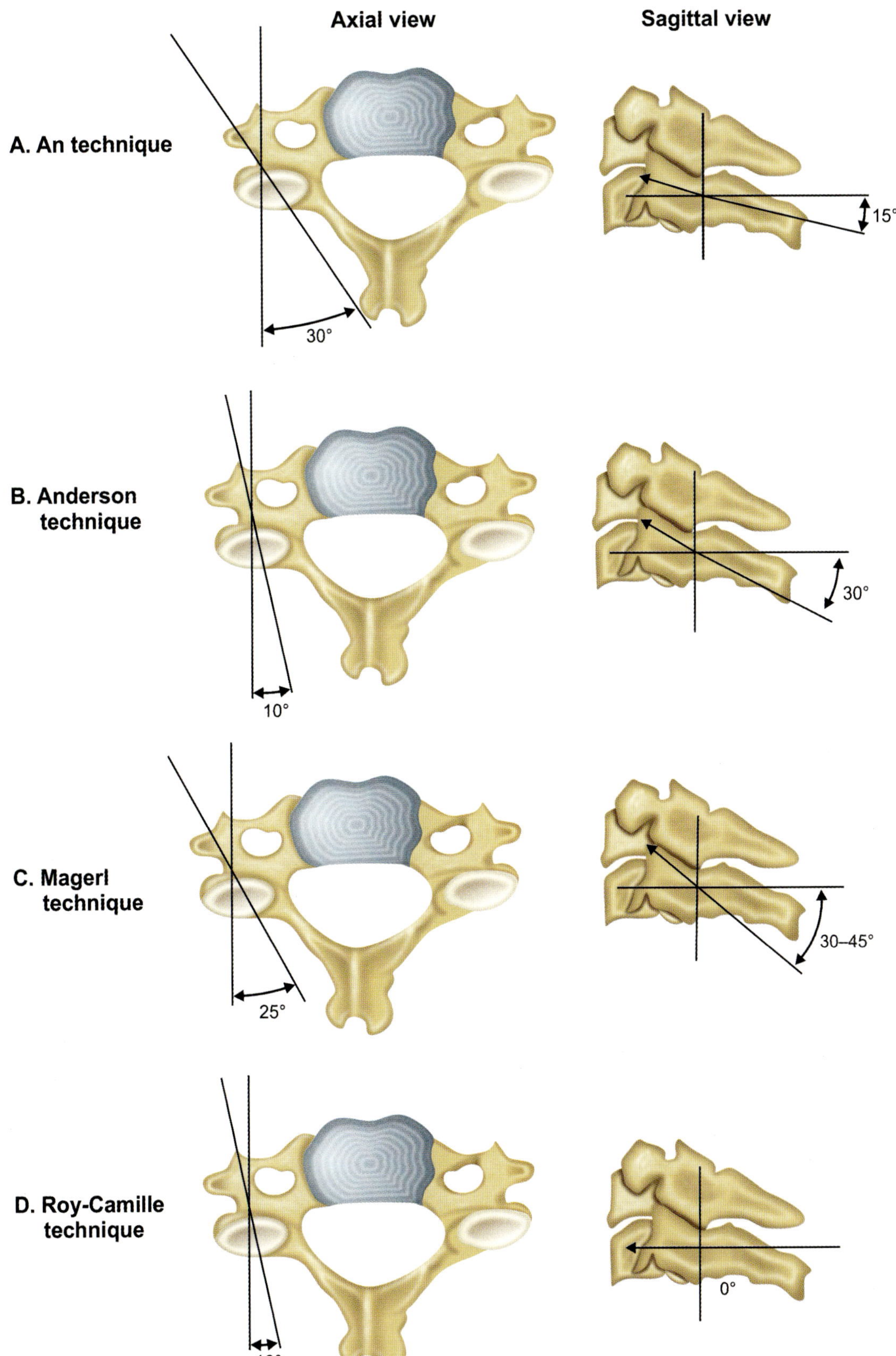

Figs. 4.13A to D: Illustrations of the screw trajectory utilized in the An (A), Anderson (B), Magerl (C), and Roy-Camille techniques (D).

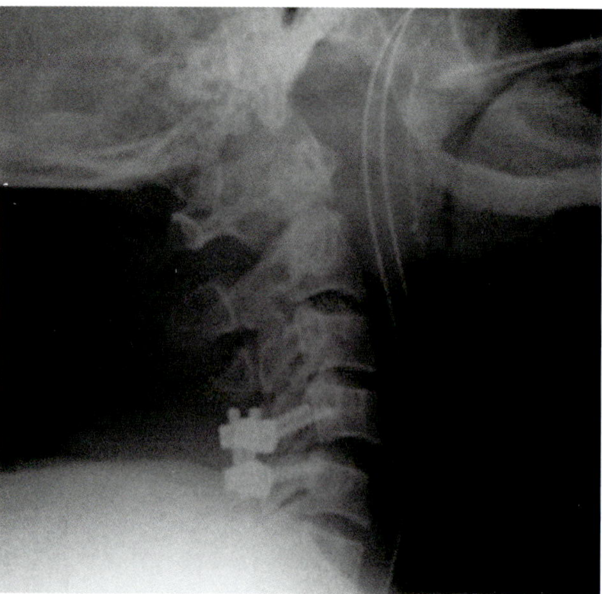

Fig. 4.14: Postoperative lateral radiograph after C4–C5 posterior cervical fusion with lateral mass screws and rod construct.

- Step 3
  - After confirming the K-wire placement, the smaller of the two cannulated cancellous drills is utilized to drill the entire length.
    - The drill diameter should be equal to the minor diameter of the screw.
  - A second drill, equal to the major diameter of the screw, is then advanced only through the superiorlateral mass.
    - In this fashion, a screw is used to lag the two segments.
- Step 4: (Figs. 4.15A and B)
  - A 7–10-mm cancellous screw can then be inserted.

GENERAL POSTOPERATIVE CARE FOR POSTERIOR MIS CERVICAL C1–C2 FUSION, SUBAXIAL LAMINECTOMY AND SUBAXIAL FUSION

Complications

- Superficial wound infections
  - Most resolve with oral antibiotics.
  - If necessary, the wound can be formally irrigated and debrided.
  - Consider intraincisional vancomycin powder for high-risk patients.
- Incidental durotomy
  - If noted intraoperatively, the durotomy can be covered with either muscle, fat, or gel foam followed by a fibrin glue or synthetic sealant.
  - For larger lacerations, a lumbar cerebrospinal fluid (CSF) diverting drain should be placed for 2–3 days to prevent a wound leak.
  - Chances of a postoperative pseudomeningocele and CSF-cutaneous fistula are rare due to the minimal dead space around the surgical site.

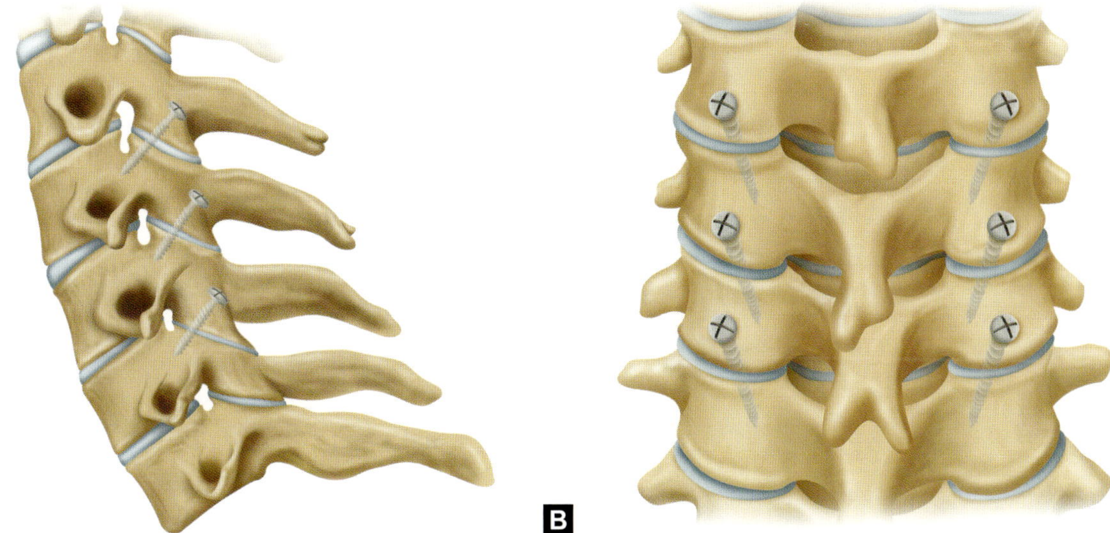

Figs. 4.15A and B: Lateral (A) and posterior (B) representation of ideal starting point and trajectory for subaxial cervical transfacet screws.

- Persistent or new axial neck pain
- Postlaminectomy kyphosis
- Segmental instability
- Inadequate decompression
- Violation of adjacent facet joint—extension of fusion into unintended levels.
- Iatrogenic fracture (lateral mass or facet)
- Vertebral artery injuries
- Pseudarthrosis

Complication Pearls

- If pulsatile bleeding is encountered from the drill hole, hemostasis can be achieved with bone wax, thrombogenic agents, and screw placement. CT angiography should be performed to determine the status of the injured vertebral artery.

Expected and Adverse Outcomes

- Short-term outcomes include a comparable patient satisfaction to that of open procedures with the added benefit of a minimally invasive approach. Some surgeons suggest that if the goals of each procedure are clearly met from a technical standpoint, there is no reason to anticipate a difference in long-term outcomes when compared with the traditional open approach.[6]
- The rate of a vertebral artery injury during C1–C2 lateral mass screw placement is 0–2.5%. The risk factors for a vertebral artery injury include direct injury due to poor screw trajectory, extended dissection along the C1 arch, or rod malposition causing intermittent compression of the vertebral artery.[7]
- A minimally invasive cervical laminectomy is well tolerated by most patients with reduced pain, shorter hospitalization, and a faster recovery.[8,9]
- Minimally invasive posterior subaxial cervical fusions are associated with a low complication rate, reduced blood loss, shorter hospitalization, and demonstrate a high fusion rate after 2 years.[10,11]
- Percutaneous posterior cervical transfacet screw placement may help reduce the risk of pseudarthrosis after a long segment anterior decompression and fusion. This technique enables a high screw pullout strength due to the penetration of four cortices.[5]

REFERENCES

1. Vaccaro AR, Baron EM. Spine surgery. Operative techniques. Philadelphia, PA: Saunders/Elsevier; 2008: 153.
2. Harms J, Melcher RP. Posterior C1-C2 fusion with polyaxial screw and rod fixation. Spine. 2001;26:2467-71.
3. Stemper BD, Marawar SV, Yoganandan N, Shender BS, Rao RD. Quantitative anatomy of subaxial cervical lateral mass: an analysis of safe screw lengths for Roy-Camille and Magerl techniques. Spine [Phila Pa 1976]. 2008;33(8):893-7.
4. Xu R, Haman SP, Ebraheim NA, Yeasting RA. The anatomic relation of lateral mass screws to the spinal nerves. A comparison of the Magerl, Anderson, and An techniques. Spine. 1999;24:2057-61.
5. Ahmad F, Sherman JD, Wang MY. Percutaneous trans-facet screws for supplemental posterior cervical fixation. World Neurosurg. 2012;78:716.e711-4.
6. Joseffer SS, Post N, Cooper PR, Frempong-Boadu AK. Minimally invasive atlantoaxial fixation with a polyaxial screw-rod construct: technical case report. Neurosurgery 2006;58:ONS-E375; discussion ONS-E375.
7. Terterov S, Taghva A, Khalessi AA, Hsieh PC. Symptomatic vertebral artery compression by the rod of a C1-C2 posterior fusion construct: case report and review of the literature. Spine (Phila Pa 1976). 2011;36:E678-1.
8. Winder MJ, Thomas KC. Minimally invasive versus open approach for cervical laminoforaminotomy. Can J Neurol Sci. 2011;38:262-7.
9. Yabuki S, Kikuchi S. Endoscopic partial laminectomy for cervical myelopathy. J Neurosurg Spine. 2005;2:170-4.
10. Wang MY, Levi AD. Minimally invasive lateral mass screw fixation in the cervical spine: initial clinical experience with long-term follow-up. Neurosurgery. 2006; 58:907-12; discussion 907-912.
11. Mikhael MM, Celestre PC, Wolf CF, Mroz TE, Wang JC. Minimally invasive cervical spine foraminotomy and lateral mass screw placement. Spine (Phila Pa 1976). 2012;37:E318-22.
12. Taghva A, et al. Minimally invasive posterior atlantoxial fusion: a cadaveric and clinical feasibility study. World Neurosurg. 2012.

REFERENCE SUMMARY

1-4, 7-9: Possible sources for Images

5. Ahmad F, Sherman JD, Wang MY. Percutaneous trans-facet screws for supplemental posterior cervical fixation. World Neurosurgery 2012;78:716 e711-4.
   Summary: Cervical transfacet screw placement is a technically feasible option in the subaxial cervical spine for spinal fixation. However, the authors recommend that until percutaneous bony fusion methods are developed, this approach should be limited to supplement an anterior fusion construct.
6. Joseffer SS, Post N, Cooper PR, Frempong-Boadu AK. Minimally invasive atlantoaxial fixation with a polyaxial screw-rod construct: technical case report. Neurosurgery 2006;58:ONS-E375; discussion ONS-E375.
   Summary: Atlantoaxial stabilization utilizing an individual fixation of the C1-lateral mass and C2 pedicle with minipolyaxial screws and rods is a safe and effective alternative to traditional open techniques.
10. Wang MY, Levi AD. Minimally invasive lateral mass screw fixation in the cervical spine: initial clinical experience with long-term follow-up. Neurosurgery 2006;58:907-912; discussion 907-12.
   Summary: Retrospective analysis of 18 patients who underwent a minimally invasive lateral mass screw placement with a 2-year follow-up. With a 100% fusion rate and no complications, the authors conclude that this approach is a safe and effective approach.
11. Mikhael MM, Celestre PC, Wolf CF, Mroz TE, Wang JC. Minimally invasive cervical spine foraminotomy and lateral mass screw placement. Spine (Phila Pa 1976) 2012;37:E318-322.
   Summary: A multilevel decompression and fusion can be safely achieved as long as the clinical outcomes are comparable with those of the conventional procedures.
12. Taghva A, et al. Minimally invasive posterior atlantoxial fusion: a cadaveric and clinical feasibility study. World Neurosurg. 2012.
   Summary: Study describes in cadavers the anatomic and fluoroscopic considerations for placement of C1 and C2 posterior cervical screws.

Chapter

5

Percutaneous Pedicle Screw Placement

Alejandro Marquez-Lara, Thomas D Cha, Kern Singh

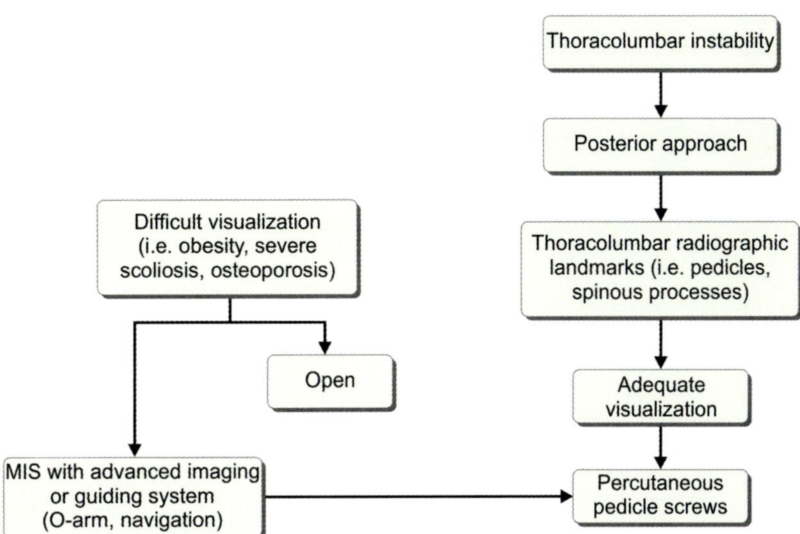

CASE VIGNETTE

A 65-year-old man with a previous history of lung cancer presents to the emergency department with acute back pain and inability to stand secondary to pain that began 6 weeks prior to presentation. On examination, the patient demonstrates tenderness over the 4th and 5th lumbar vertebrae.

DIAGNOSTIC IMAGING

- Plain film radiograph—Anteroposterior (AP) and lateral
  - Initial plain films provide an early assessment of the fracture pattern and stability.
- Computed tomography (CT) (Figs. 5.1A to C)
  - Reconstruction in the sagittal and coronal plane will define the fracture pattern and assist with preoperative planning.
    - For each pedicle screw, the maximum diameter (in particular the transverse diameter) and the length should be measured.
  - Images can be utilized intraoperatively with advanced image guidance systems.

Imaging Pearls

- Intrapedicular distance should be evaluated to determine if there is bony destruction.
- The spinous process alignment should be evaluated to determine if bony destruction has occurred.

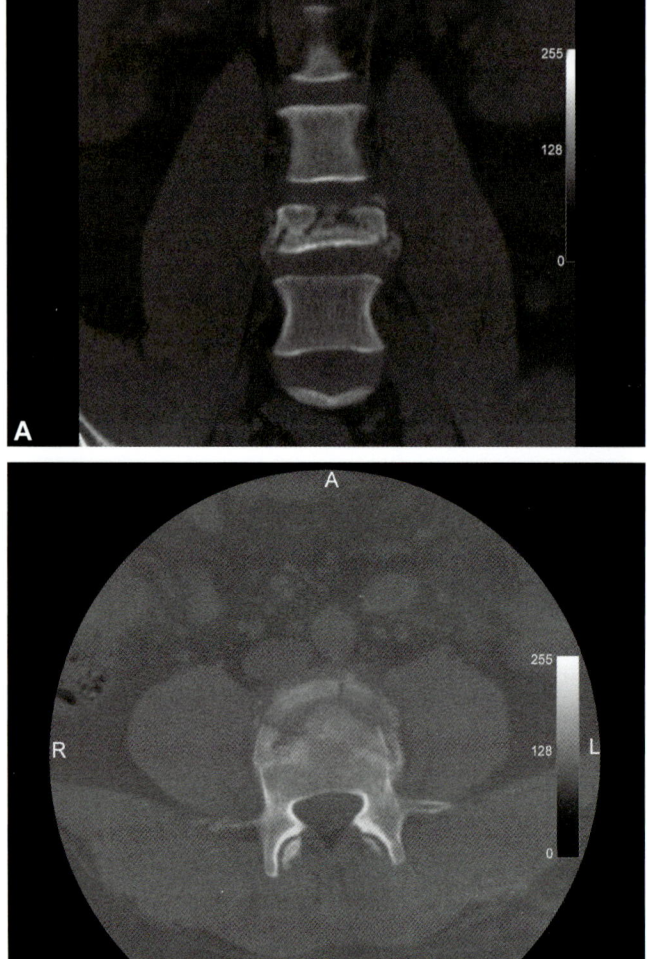

Figs. 5.1A to C: Preoperative (A) coronal, (B) sagittal, and (C) axial computer tomography of the lumbar spine demonstrating a pathologic fracture at the L4 body.

- Magnetic resonance imaging (MRI)
  - If there is concern for spinal cord compression or injury, an MRI is indicated to assess the spinal cord and the surrounding soft tissues.
  - Screw diameter and length can also be measured from the axial MRI images.

SURGICAL INDICATIONS

- Thoracic/lumbar spine instability
  - Trauma
    - Flexion-distraction injury
    - Unstable burst fractures
    - Initial stabilization of a polytraumatized patient

Indication Pearls

- In patients with neurological compromise, percutaneous screws can be combined with an anterior or posterior decompression.

Contraindications

- Inability to adequately identify the radiographic anatomic landmarks in two planes.

Controversies

- In patients who are obese or osteoporotic an intraoperative navigation system can help identify critical landmarks for percutaneous pedicle screw placement.

- Pathologic fractures
  - Metastatic disease
  - Osteoporotic
- Degenerative conditions
  - Spondylolisthesis
  - Scoliosis
- Neoplasia
- Infection

INSTRUMENTATION

- Radiolucent table
- Intraoperative fluoroscopy with or without navigation
  - C-arm
  - O-arm
- Spinal access needle
  - Jamshidi needle or a sharp-tipped pedicle awl
- Pedicle tap
- Percutaneous pedicle screw instrumentation

Instrumentation Pearls

- Cement augmentation (kyphoplasty/vertebroplasty) is sometimes utilized in combination with percutaneous pedicle screw fixation.

Positioning and Intraoperative Setup

- Neuromonitoring with somatosensory and motor-evoked potentials should be utilized for purposes of positioning.
- The patient is placed into a prone position on a radiolucent table.
  - Appropriate padding is placed over bony prominences.
  - Chest and hip pads are adjusted to increase or decrease thoracic kyphosis.
- Fluoroscopy should be positioned over the trunk of the patient.
  - Intraoperative fluoroscopy is of particular importance during this procedure to determine the trajectory and the entry points for the pedicle screws.
  - Confirmation of the pedicle image should be done both in the AP and lateral planes.
    - The fluoroscopic projection should be parallel to the end plates at the level of the screw insertion (Fig. 5.2).

Surgical Anatomy and Exposure

- Relevant anatomy
  - The thoracic pedicle has a greater vertical than transverse diameter (T4 has the smallest diameter).
    - Screw size should be 0.5 mm smaller than the transverse diameter of the pedicle.
  - The medial wall of the thoracic pedicle is thicker than the lateral wall.
  - The thoracic pedicles have a decreasing medial angulation in the transverse plane from T1 (~30°) to T12 (~7°). In the sagittal plane, the pedicles have a 10°–20° cephalad angulation.

Exposure Pearls

- The spinous process should be midline between the pedicles in a true direct AP view.

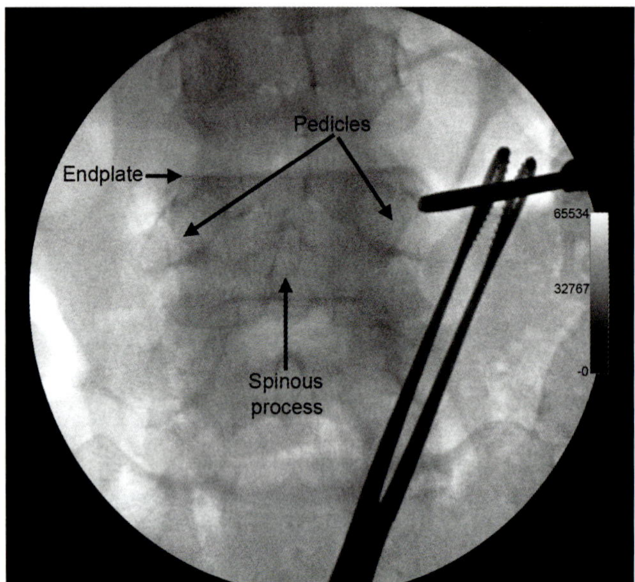

Fig. 5.2: An intraoperative radiograph depicting critical anatomic landmarks. The endplate is seen as a single solid line, which confirms adequate fluoroscopic projection.

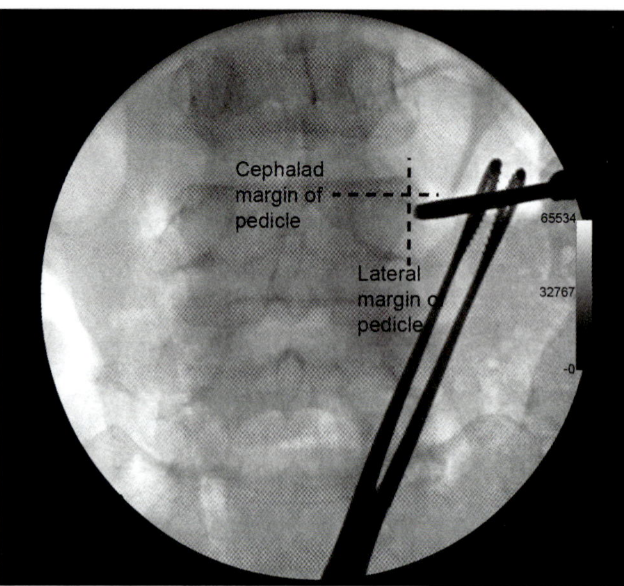

Fig. 5.3: An anteroposterior intraoperative fluoroscopy depicting the intersection of the cephalad and lateral margin of the pedicle, which can help guide the site for the skin incision.

- The lumbar pedicles have an increasing medial angulation in the transverse plane from L1 (5°–10°) to L5 (20°–30°). In the sagittal plane, the lumbar pedicles have a relatively shallow caudal angulation between 2° and 10°.

PROCEDURE-SPECIFIC STEPS

- Step 1
  - After identifying the level of interest, a 10-mm longitudinal skin incision is made 10-20 mm laterally to the midline along the lateral edge of the lateral pedicle wall.
    - The intersection of the cephalad and lateral margin of the pedicle in the AP view can be utilized as a guide for the skin incision (Fig. 5.3).
  - A spinal access needle (Jamshidi needle or a sharp-tipped pedicle awl) is angled medially and placed at the intersection of the lateral border of the superior facet and a bisecting line of the transverse process.
- Step 2
  - The spinal access needle is advanced with a gentle twisting motion into the pedicle or with the aid of a hammer. The Jamshidi should be advanced in increments of 5 mm until the tip is centered in the pedicle (15–20 mm) (Fig. 5.4).
  - Care should be taken to not violate any of the pedicle borders.
    - If the Jamshidi tip is crossing the medial wall on the pedicle prior to 15 mm of depth then the starting point should be re-evaluated as a medial wall breech is likely.

Procedure Pitfalls

- Percutaneous thoracic fixation exposes the surgeon and the patient to a higher dose of radiation due to the greater fluoroscopy time needed for screw placement.

Step 1 Pearls

- In obese patients, the skin incision should be more lateral to achieve an adequate alignment of the spinal needle within the pedicles.
- The correct starting position of the Jamshidi needle is at the lateral margin of the pedicle.
  - 2 o'clock on the right pedicle
  - 10 o'clock on the left pedicle
- The starting point can vary slightly between the different levels of the thoracic spine.

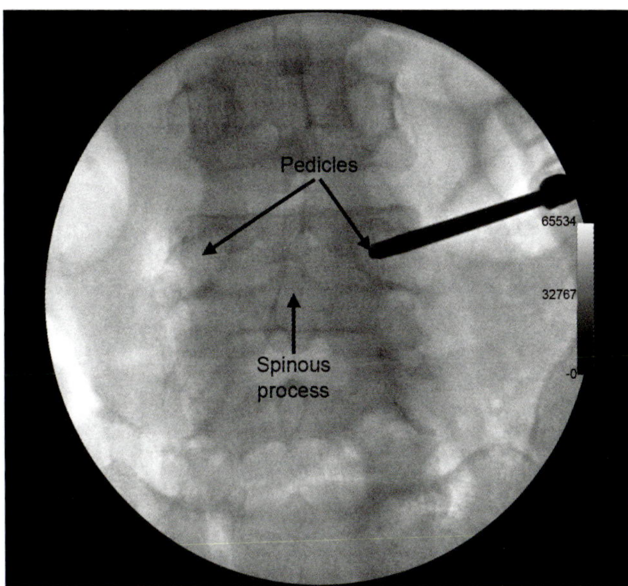

Fig. 5.4: Intraoperative radiograph demonstrating the spinal access needle centered on the pedicle in the anteroposterior projection.

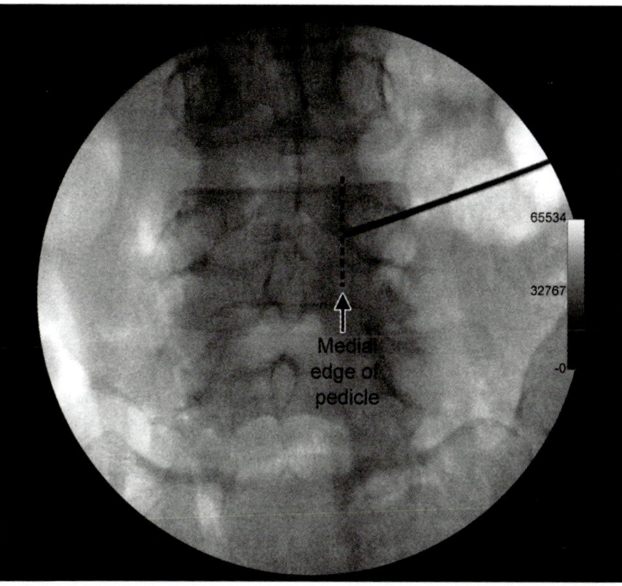

Fig. 5.5: Anteroposterior intraoperative radiograph demonstrating appropriate guidewire position. Note how the guidewire is not crossing the medial edge of the pedicle.

- Step 3
  - A guidewire is then inserted through the Jamshidi, an additional 10–15 mm until it just crosses the medial wall of the pedicle on the AP plane (Fig. 5.5).
  - A lateral view is then obtained confirming that the guidewire is in the vertebral body.
    - If the guidewire has not reached the vertebral body on the lateral plane then a medial wall violation has occurred.
    - Over penetration of the guidewire can perforate the anterior cortex of the vertebral body and potentially injure the great vessels and viscera.
  - The spinal access needle is then carefully removed over the guidewire, and the procedure should be repeated for the adjacent levels (Figs. 5.6A and B).
- Step 4
  - A small fascial incision is made centered around each of the guidewires and sequential soft tissue dilation is performed to allow for further instrumentation.
- Step 5
  - A pedicle tap is then advanced over the guidewire to prepare the pedicles for screw placement (Fig. 5.7).
    - The tap should be at least 0.5 mm smaller than the anticipated screw size.
    - The tap can be stimulated and electromyography evoked responses can be utilized to determine if there is a medial wall breach.

Step 3 Pearls

- If the surgeon is unable to appreciate the anatomical landmarks or there is a concern for a possible screw breakout, a bull's-eye view should be obtained of the pedicle. The Jamshidi needle should be centered within the pedicle on the bull's-eye view.

Procedure Pitfalls

- Inadvertent guidewire advancement can occur when tapping is not aligned with the guidewire trajectory.

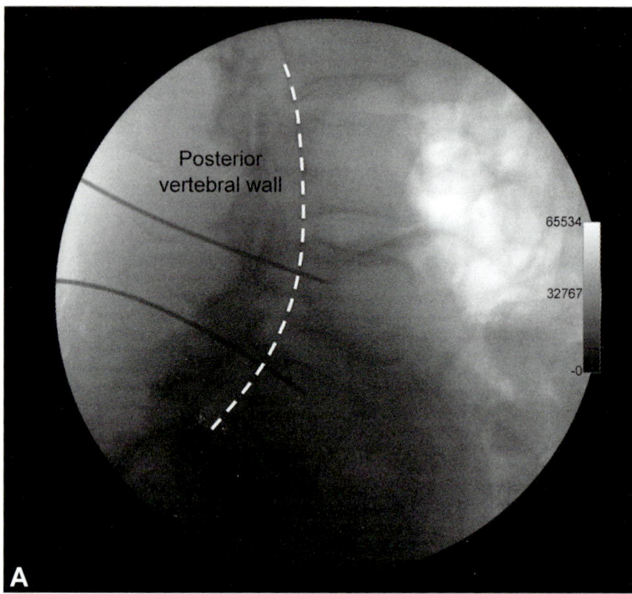

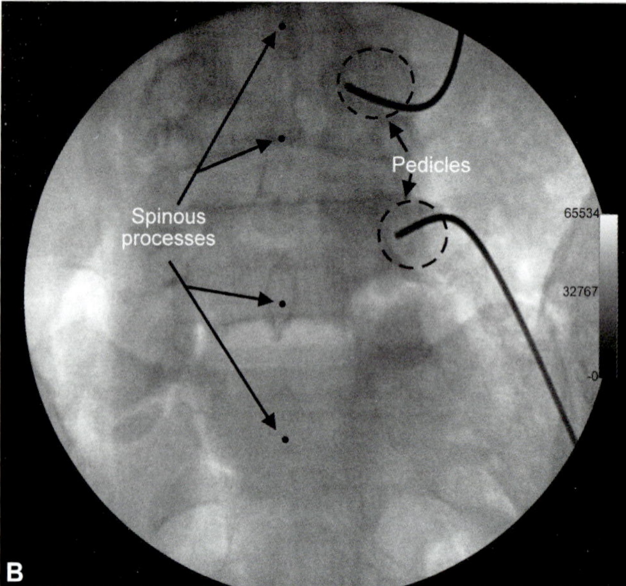

Figs. 5.6A and B: The same radiographic technique is utilized to access the pedicles at the adjacent level. The guidewires are positioned well past the posterior wall of the vertebral body (A) while preserving the integrity of the pedicles (B).

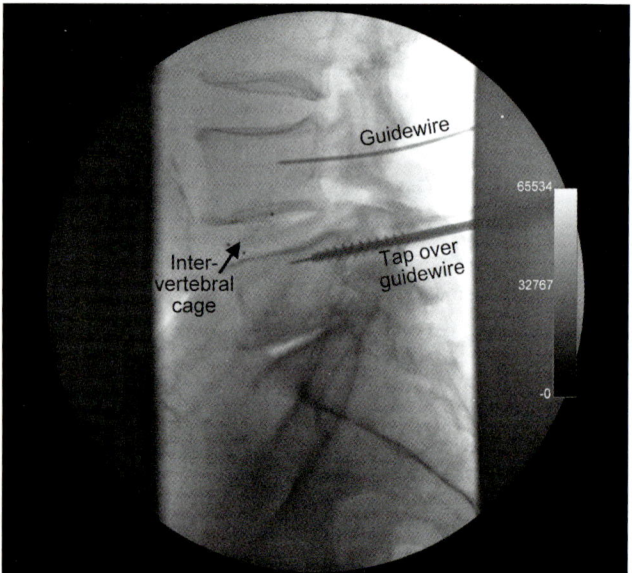

Fig. 5.7: Lateral fluoroscopy demonstrating a pedicle tap placed over the guidewire.

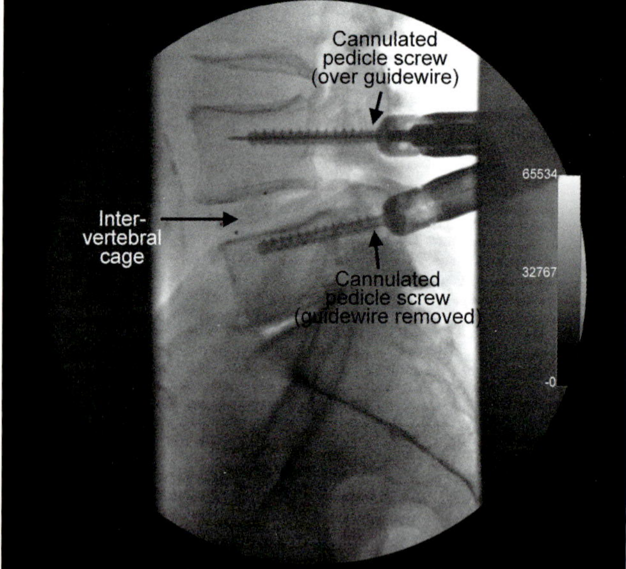

Fig. 5.8: An intraoperative radiograph demonstrating two cannulated pedicle screws placed over guidewires.

- Step 6
  - The tap is removed over the guidewire, and a cannulated pedicle screw of the appropriate length and diameter is then inserted under fluoroscopic guidance (Fig. 5.8).
  - After screw placement, an AP and lateral fluoroscopic view should be obtained to assess the screw positioning.

Step 6 Pearls

- The final screw placement should be parallel to superior end plate.

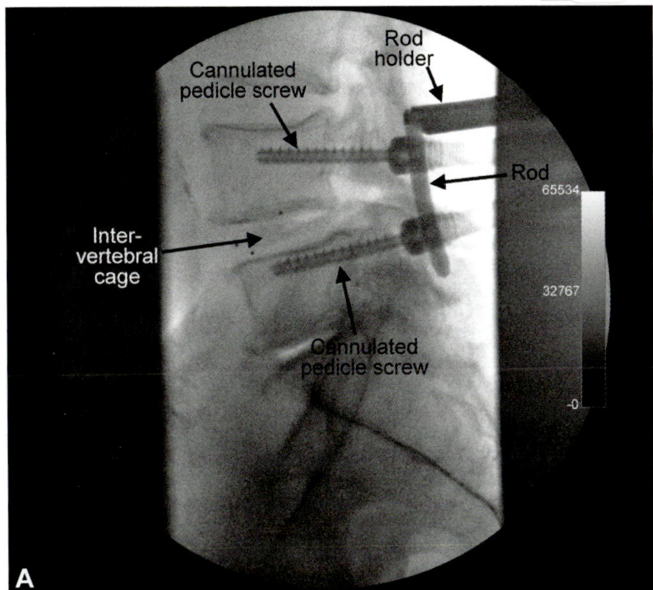

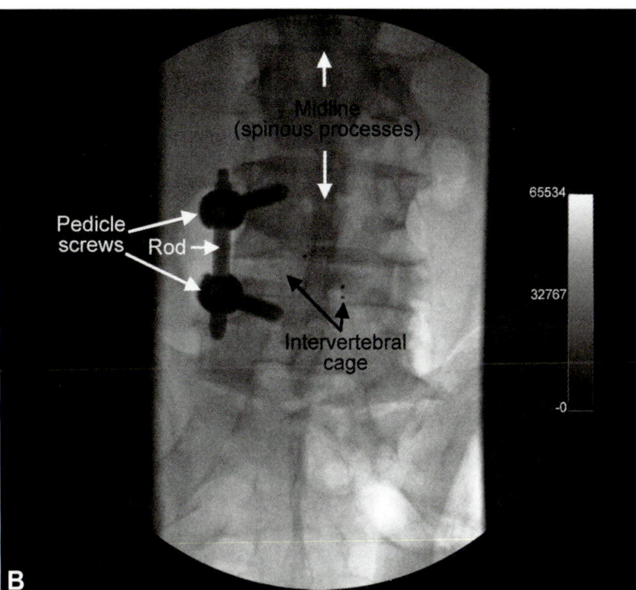

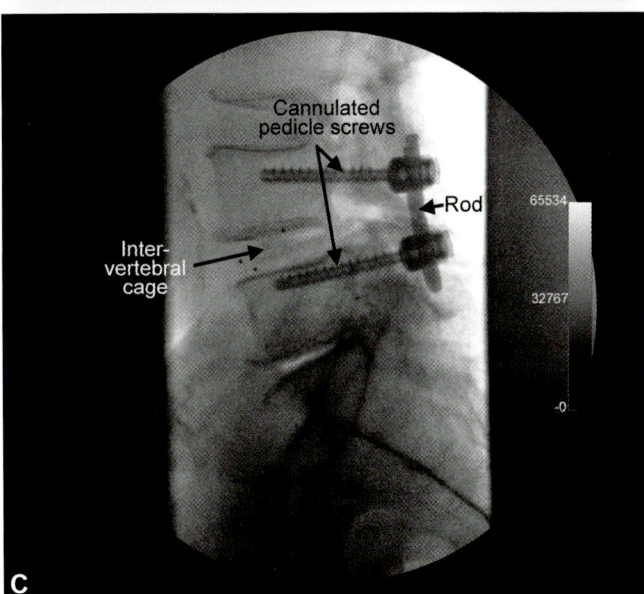

Figs. 5.9A to C: An intraoperative lateral radiograph demonstrating the insertion of a submuscular rod into the tulips of the pedicle screws (A). The final construct is assessed with anteroposterior (B) and lateral radiographs (C).

- Step 7
  - The pedicle screw extenders are then lined up to allow the rod to pass through the slots (Figs. 5.9A to C).
    - Lateral fluoroscopic imaging confirms the appropriate length and depth of the rod.

Step 7 Pearls

- Appropriate depth of screw insertion can be gauged by the height of the screw extenders, which also can serve as a guide for rod contouring.

POSTOPERATIVE CARE

Complications

- Although rare, pedicle screw malposition can result in the following:
  - Nerve root injury
  - Spinal cord injury

- Vascular injury
- Visceral injury
- Screw pullout

EXPECTED AND ADVERSE OUTCOMES

- With experienced hands, percutaneous transpedicular instrumentation is an accurate, reliable, and safe method to address spinal instability.[1,2]
- Percutaneous pedicle screw fixation is technically possible and safe in a variety of thoracic spinal disorders with conventional two-dimensional fluoroscopy alone.[3] However, this procedure is technically demanding with potential risk of injury to the spinal cord and the great vessels.[4]
- Fluoroscopy-assisted pedicle screw insertion is associated with less pedicle wall violation when compared with an open surgery at the expense of greater radiation exposure.[5,6] Other advantages of percutaneous pedicle screw fixation include the preservation of posterior musculature, less blood loss, shorter operative time, lower infection risk, less postoperative pain, and a shorter hospital stay.[6]

REFERENCES

1. Heintel TM, Berglehner A, Meffert R. Accuracy of percutaneous pedicle screws for thoracic and lumbar spine fractures: a prospective trial. Eur Spine J: official publication of the European Spine Society, the European Spinal Deformity Society, and the European Section of the Cervical Spine Research Society. 2013;22:495-502.
2. Raley DA, Mobbs RJ. Retrospective computed tomography scan analysis of percutaneously inserted pedicle screws for posterior transpedicular stabilization of the thoracic and lumbar spine: accuracy and complication rates. Spine (Phila Pa 1976). 2012;37:1092-1100.
3. Ringel F, Stoffel M, Stuer C, Meyer B. Minimally invasive transmuscular pedicle screw fixation of the thoracic and lumbar spine. Neurosurgery. 2006;59:ONS361-366; discussion ONS366-367.
4. Hu HT, Shin JH, Hwang JY, et al. Thoracic aortic stent-graft placement for safe removal of a malpositioned pedicle screw. Cardiovasc Intervent Radiol. 2010;33:1040-3.
5. Wild MH, Glees M, Plieschnegger C, Wenda K. Five-year follow-up examination after purely minimally invasive posterior stabilization of thoracolumbar fractures: a comparison of minimally invasive percutaneously and conventionally open treated patients. Arch Orthop Trauma Surg. 2007;127:335-43.
6. Court C, Vincent C. Percutaneous fixation of thoracolumbar fractures: current concepts. Orthop Traumatol Surg Res: OTSR. 2012;98:900-09.

REFERENCE SUMMARY

1. Heintel TM, Berglehner A, Meffert R. Accuracy of percutaneous pedicle screws for thoracic and lumbar spine fractures: a prospective trial. European spine journal : official publication of the European Spine Society, the European Spinal Deformity Society, and the European Section of the Cervical Spine Research Society 2013;22:495-502.

   Summary: A prospective study of 502 pedicle screws placed in 111 patients with conventional fluoroscopy. The authors demonstrated that 85% of the screws were classified as good to excellent in length, and 98% were classified as good to excellent in position.

2. Raley DA, Mobbs RJ. Retrospective computed tomography scan analysis of percutaneously inserted pedicle screws for posterior transpedicular stabilization of the thoracic and lumbar spine: accuracy and complication rates. Spine (Phila Pa 1976) 2012;37:1092-1100.

Summary: 90.3% of 424 percutaneously inserted thoracolumbar pedicle screws were placed without pedicle breakout. This technique is an acceptable option with a low complication rate in experienced hands.

5. Wild MH, Glees M, Plieschnegger C, Wenda K. Five-year follow-up examination after purely minimally invasive posterior stabilization of thoracolumbar fractures: a comparison of minimally invasive percutaneously and conventionally open treated patients. Archives of Orthopaedic and Trauma Surgery 2007;127:335-43.

Summary: A 5-year follow-up of 21 patients who underwent an open or percutaneous thoracolumbar fixation for type-A fractures. Clinical and radiological outcomes were similar between the cohorts. However, the percutaneous cohort demonstrated less intraoperative blood loss at the cost of greater radiation exposure.

6. Court C, Vincent C. Percutaneous fixation of thoracolumbar fractures: current concepts. Orthopaedics & Traumatology, Surgery & Research: OTSR 2012;98:900-909.

Summary: The authors present a thorough review of the current treatment advantages and disadvantages of percutaneous posterior thoracic pedicle screw placement. Larger prospective trials are necessary to clarify the indications for this minimally invasive technique.

Chapter

6

Minimally Invasive Lateral Retropleural Approach for Thoracic Discectomy and Corpectomy

Kern Singh, Sreeharsha V Nandyala, Damandeep Singh Makkar, Alexander R Vaccaro

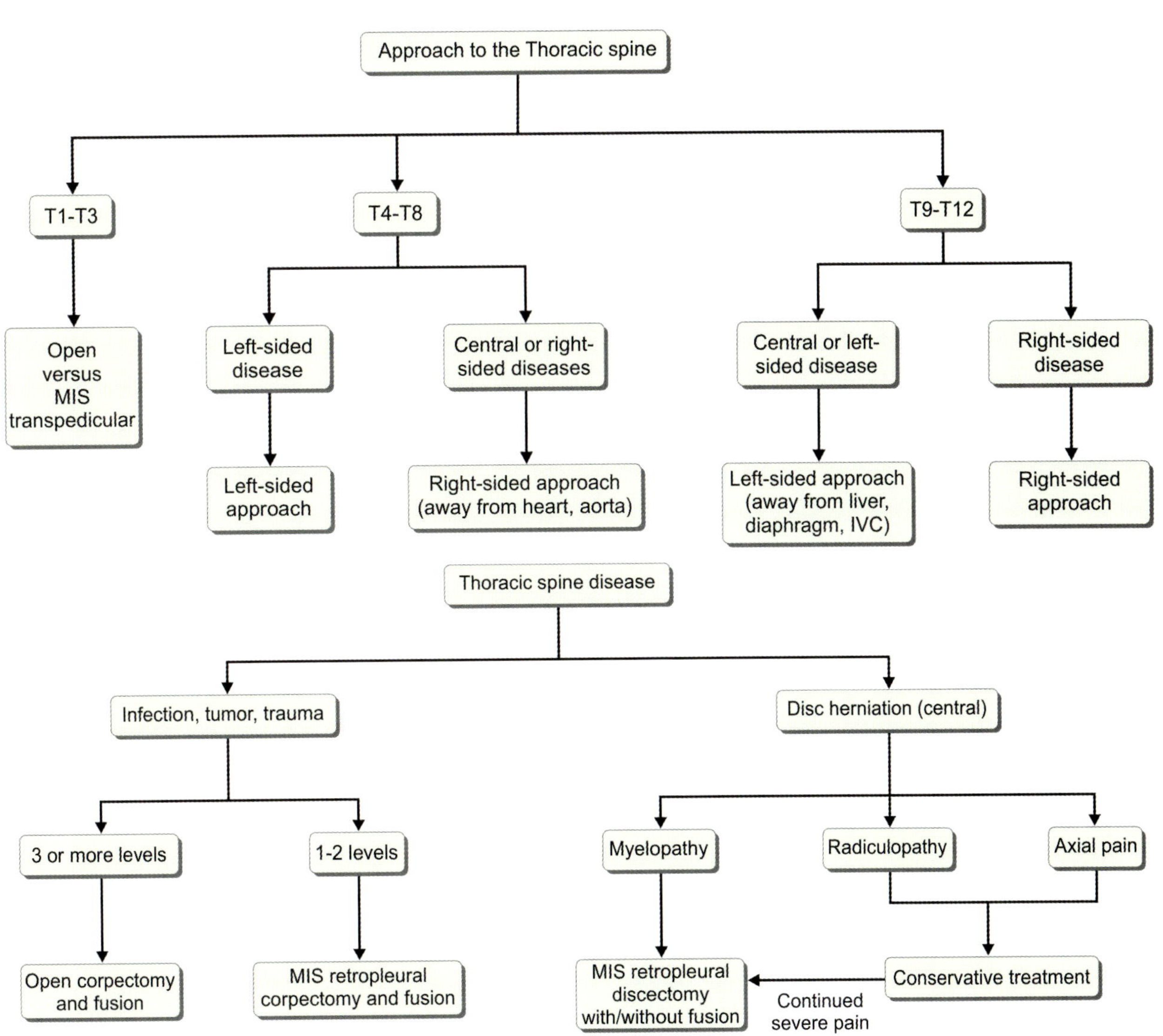

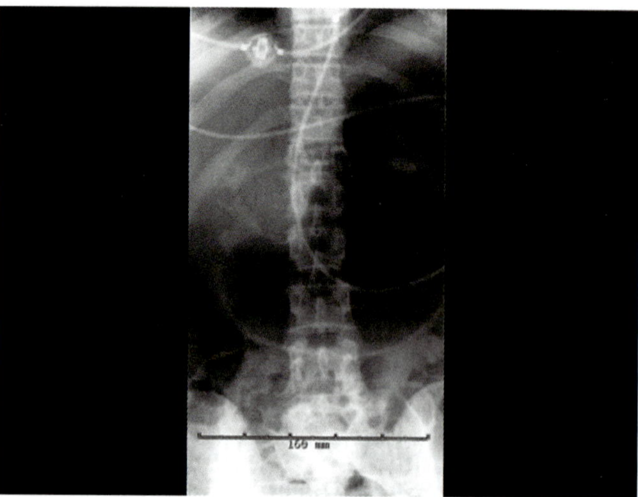

Fig. 6.1: Preoperative anteroposterior demonstrating vertebral body collapse at T12.

CASE VIGNETTE

A 47-year-old woman presents to the office with worsening upper back pain, gait disturbance, and intermittent lower extremity weakness. She denies recent trauma or bowel and bladder dysfunction. On examination, the patient demonstrates hyper-reflexia and spasticity of the right lower extremity. The symptoms have been worsening despite physical therapy and anti-inflammatory medications.

DIAGNOSTIC IMAGING

- Plain film radiograph—Antero-posterior and lateral
  - Provides an initial assessment of the disc space, vertebral body, and stability of the thoracic spine (Fig. 6.1)
- Computed tomography (CT) (Figs. 6.2A and B)
  - Enables the assessment of the spinal cord, intervertebral disc, and helps with preoperative instrumentation templating (vertebral body size, pedicle width/length)
  - Magnetic resonance imaging (MRI)
  - An MRI is the most sensitive imaging study to evaluate for spinal cord compression and the extent of intervertebral disc pathology (Fig. 6.3).
    - A gadolinium-enhanced MRI should be obtained if there is concern for a neoplasm or infection.

SURGICAL INDICATIONS

- Tumor
  - Primary
  - Metastatic

Indication Pearls

- Rib fractures, costochondritis, cardiac disease, and cholelithiasis can mimic thoracic radicular pain.

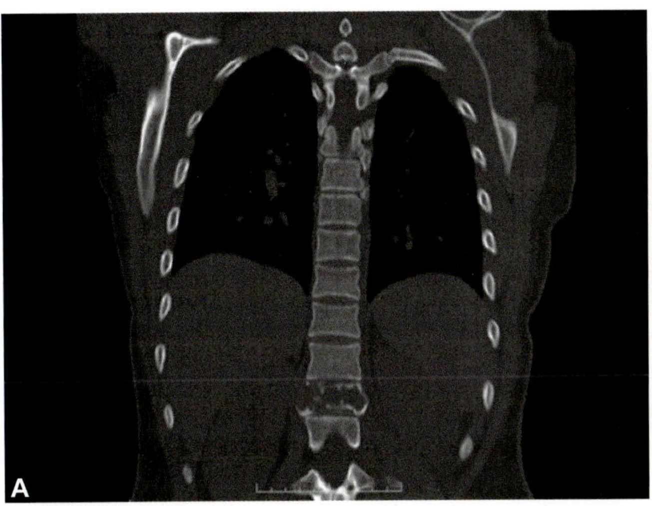

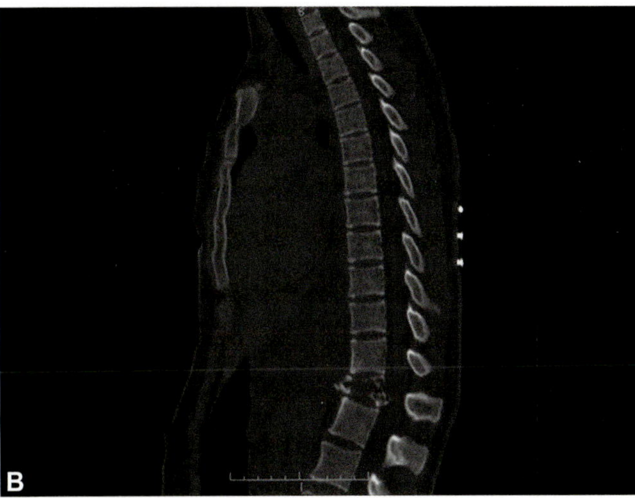

Figs. 6.2A and B: (A) Coronal and (B) sagittal preoperative computer tomography demonstrating significant T12 vertebral body destruction resulting in a kyphotic deformity.

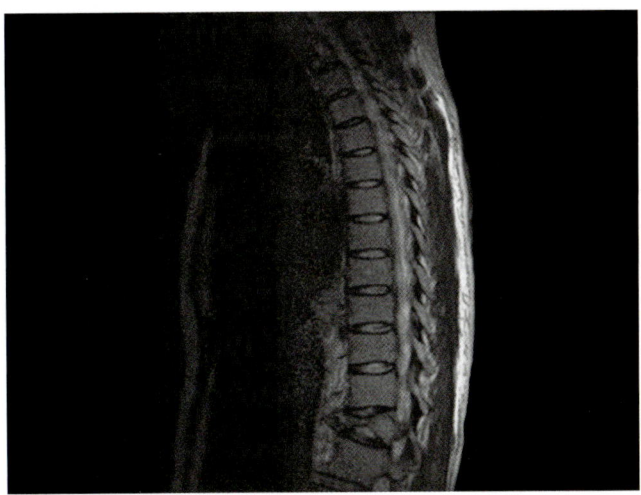

Fig. 6.3: Sagittal magnetic resonance imaging demonstrating spinal cord involvement from retropulsion of T12 vertebral body segments.

- Unstable thoracic fractures
  - Trauma
  - Pathologic
- Osteomyelitis or discitis
- Symptomatic herniated nucleus pulposus
- Deformity correction

INSTRUMENTATION

- Expandable (split-blade) retractor and table-mounted retractor arm.
- High-speed burr
- Angled curettes
- Rongeurs
- Hemostatic agents (Gelfoam, gelatin sponge, bone wax)
- Intraoperative fluoroscopy

Contraindications

- Prior thoracotomy on the side of access (because of the likelihood of dense pleural adhesions)
- Severe cardiac or pulmonary disease
- Morbid obesity

Controversies

- 3+ level corpectomy
- Pathology above T6 due to the prominence of the scapula in the surgical field.

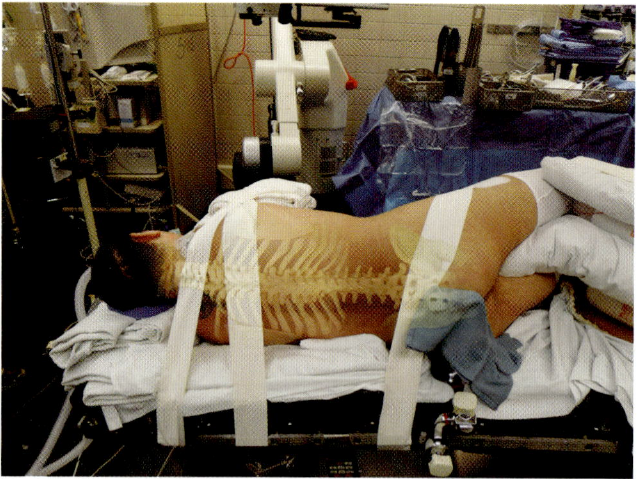

Fig. 6.4: A patient is positioned in a lateral decubitus position on a flat radiolucent table. The chest and the pelvis are stabilized perpendicular to the table.

POSITIONING AND INTRAOPERATIVE SETUP

- Endotracheal intubation is performed in a supine position.
  - A double-lumen endotracheal tube is utilized for optional single-lung ventilation during the procedure.
  - A bronchial blocker can also be utilized to temporarily deflate the ipsilateral lung during exposure.
- Neuromonitoring with somatosensory and motor-evoked potentials should be utilized.
- The patient is placed in a lateral decubitus position. (Fig. 6.4).
  - A left-lateral decubitus position for a right-sided approach is preferred for the upper thoracic spine (T4–T9) to avoid the arch and descending aorta.
  - A right-lateral decubitus position for a left-sided approach is preferred in the lower thoracic levels (T10–L2) to avoid the liver and the diaphragm.
- Appropriate padding is placed over the bony prominences.
- An axillary roll is positioned under the dependent axilla.
- Both arms are flexed forward.
  - Abducting the superior arm by 90°–100° displaces the scapula and shoulder girdle to reach as high as the T3 level.
- The pelvis and upper thorax are taped to enable flexion without moving the patient.
- The surgeon should be positioned posterior to the patient with the patient positioned as close to the edge of the bed as possible (toward the surgeon).
- The fluoroscopy monitor and the mounted retractor arm should be on the opposite side of the surgeon.

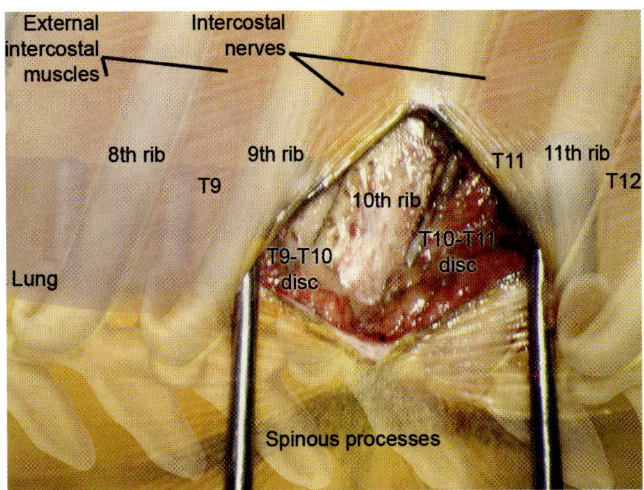

Fig. 6.5: Photograph demonstrating exposure of the rib.

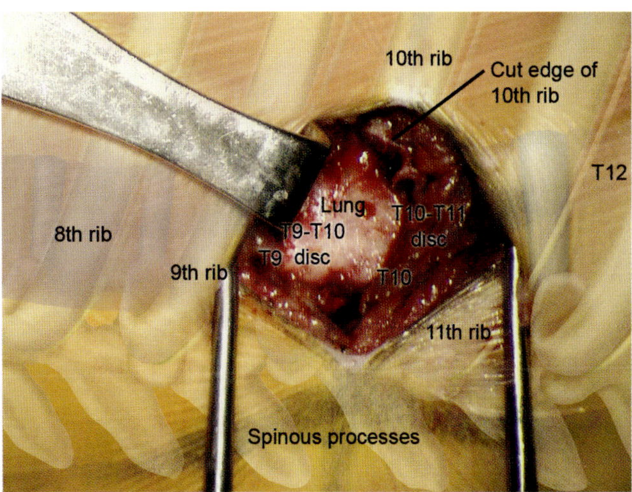

Fig. 6.6: Intraoperative photograph demonstrating the exposed parietal pleura after resecting approximately 2 cm of the overlying rib.

SURGICAL ANATOMY AND EXPOSURE

- Relevant anatomy
  - The thoracic aorta lies ventral to the spine and demarcates the ventral border of the vertebral column.
  - The ventral (or segmental) branch of the intercostal artery supplies the vertebral bodies. The artery runs in a horizontal trajectory between the ventral nerve root and the posterior cortex of the vertebral body.
  - The thoracic duct begins on the vertebral cortex of L2, medial to the aorta. It courses cephalad in the posterior mediastinum on the bodies of T6–T12. The thoracic aorta is to its left and the Azygos vein to its right.
  - The diaphragm inserts at the T12–L1 level.
    - In general, when working at the thoracolumbar junction a subdiaphragmatic approach is utilized to avoid the diaphragm.
- Surgical exposure
  - With lateral fluoroscopic guidance, the level of interest is localized.
  - A 30–40-mm skin incision is centered over the index vertebra and is made in-line with the superior surface of the overlying rib (Fig. 6.5).
  - The rib is exposed subperiosteally, and the neurovascular bundle is reflected inferiorly.
  - Approximately, 2 cm of the rib overlying the index vertebra is resected (Fig. 6.6).
    - This can be utilized as autologous bone graft during the procedure.
  - At this point, the parietal pleura and lung are bluntly deflected anteriorly away from the thoracic wall with a sweeping motion using a sponge stick. Dissection should be directed posteriorly along the undersurface of the rib thereby sweeping the retropleural space anteriorly.

Exposure pearls

- Resection of the rib allows for easier expansion of the retractor without concern for a rib fracture. In addition, the rib can be re-approximated at the end of surgery with a maxillofacial plate.
- Typically, a three-bladed retractor is utilized. The blades are oriented such that no blade is placed posteriorly. In this orientation, there is no blade obscuring visualization of the posterior vertebral body and spinal canal.

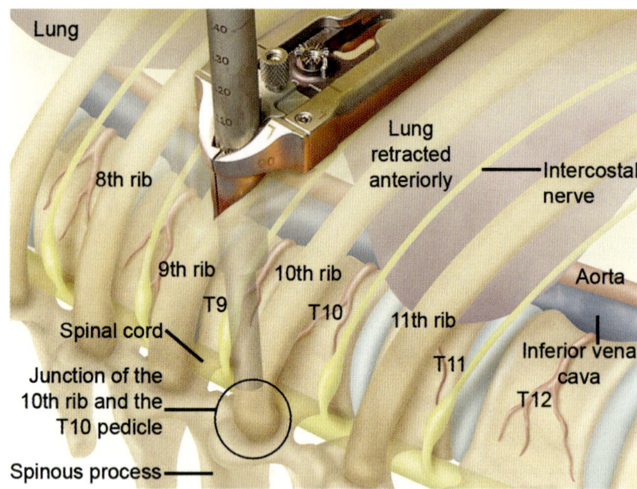

Fig. 6.7: The parietal pleura and lung are bluntly swept anteriorly, which enables the placement for sequential dilators that create a retropleural working channel and hold the lung and pleura anteriorly.

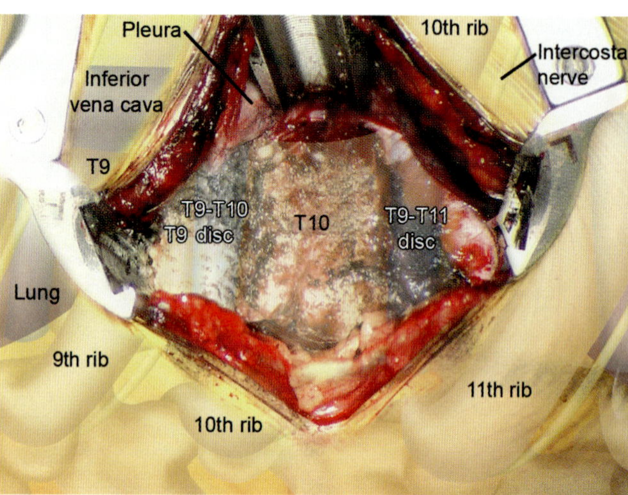

Fig. 6.8: Intraoperative photograph demonstrating a completely exposed vertebral body and adjacent disc spaces after resecting the overlying rib head.

- The initial dilator is advanced under fluoroscopic guidance and tactile feedback until it docks onto the lateral aspect of the vertebral body (rib head junction) at the level of interest.
- Sequential dilation is then performed (Fig. 6.7). After reaching the final dilator, an expandable retractor is placed over the dilators and subsequently secured onto the table-mounted retractor arm.
- After assuring visualization of the index vertebral body, the disc spaces and the vertebral bodies above and below are exposed subperiostally, and the segmental artery is cauterized and resected.
- The rib head at the corresponding vertebra is identified and resected, thereby exposing the posterior vertebral body, pedicle, and intervertebral disc (Fig. 6.8).
- The pedicle at the level of interest is resected with a high-speed burr, and a Kerrison rongeur is utilized for access to the canal. This maneuver will expose the lateral dural sac and the exiting nerve root.

PROCEDURE-SPECIFIC STEPS—THORACIC DISCECTOMY

- Step 1
  - Staying just anterior to the canal, a trough is created by drilling the posterior third of the vertebral body adjacent to the disc space and the superior half of the inferior pedicle.
- Step 2
  - The herniated disc fragments are then removed by pulling them anteriorly into the trough and avoiding any pressure on the spinal cord.
- Step 3
  - If a large portion of the vertebral body and disc are removed, a fusion should be performed utilizing the resected rib portion as autograft.

Step 1 Pearls

- Fluoroscopic imaging will provide a rough estimation of the canal and the amount of ventral vertebral body that should be resected.

Step 2 Pitfalls

- A large calcified herniated disc may be adherent to the posterior longitudinal ligament and dura, which may lead to an inadvertent durotomy.

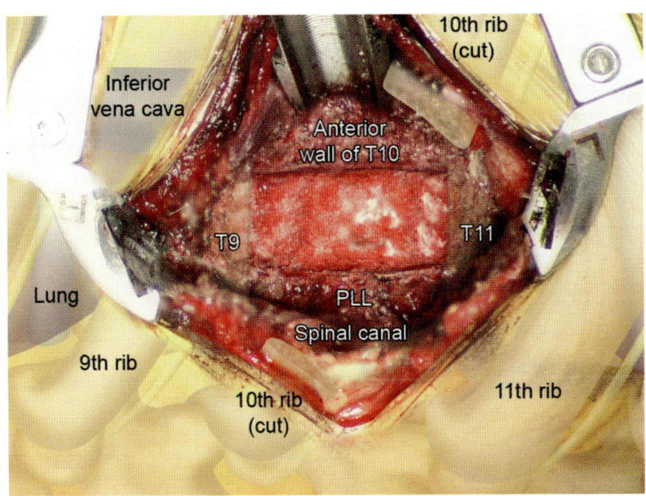

Fig. 6.9: Corpectomy and discectomy have been performed while preserving a thin portion of the anterior vertebral wall and the posterior longitudinal ligament.

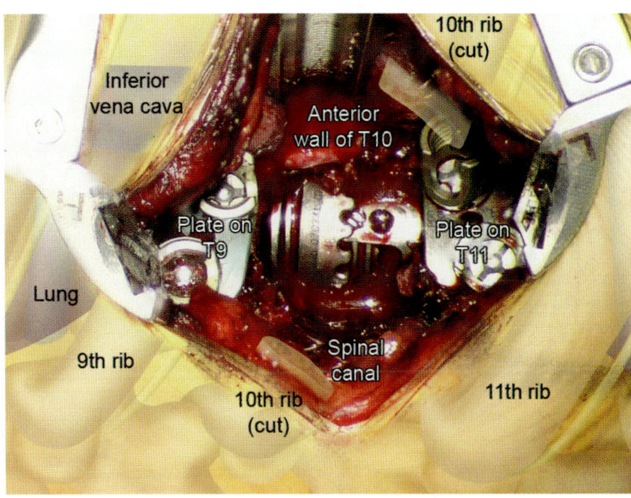

Fig. 6.10: An expandable titanium cage has been sized and inserted into the defect. Ventrolateral plates and screws have also been placed in the vertebral bodies above and below.

- Step 4
  - The surgical site is irrigated and instruments are removed.
  - After removing the retractor, the wound is closed in layers.

PROCEDURE-SPECIFIC STEPS—THORACIC CORPECTOMY

- Step 1
  - The borders of the corpectomy are defined by resecting the intervertebral discs above and below with an angled curette and a Kerrison rongeur
    - The rib head caudal to the index vertebra is resected to fully expose the inferior intervertebral disc.
- Step 2
  - The vertebral body is resected utilizing a high-speed burr, rongeurs, and curettes. Care should be taken to preserve a thin portion of the anterior cortex and the anterior longitudinal ligament (The anterior cortex is resected in cases of primary spinal tumors). (Fig. 6.9).
    - If the posterior longitudinal ligament is not part of the compressive pathology, it should be left intact.
  - Lateral fluoroscopic imaging is utilized to confirm the extent of the corpectomy.
- Step 3
  - After resecting the vertebral body, an expandable titanium cage is sized and placed into the defect for reconstruction of the vertebral body.
  - The cage is expanded under lateral fluoroscopic imaging until the desired sagittal alignment is achieved (Fig. 6.10).
  - Autologous bone graft or a substitute is placed inside the cage to promote fusion.

Step 2 Pearls

- Preservation of the posterior longitudinal ligament (PLL) in noncompressive pathology helps avoid over distraction of the spinal segment.

Step 3 Pearls

- Care is taken to pack bone graft around the cage as well. Oftentimes, the fusion mass occurs around the corpectomy cage.

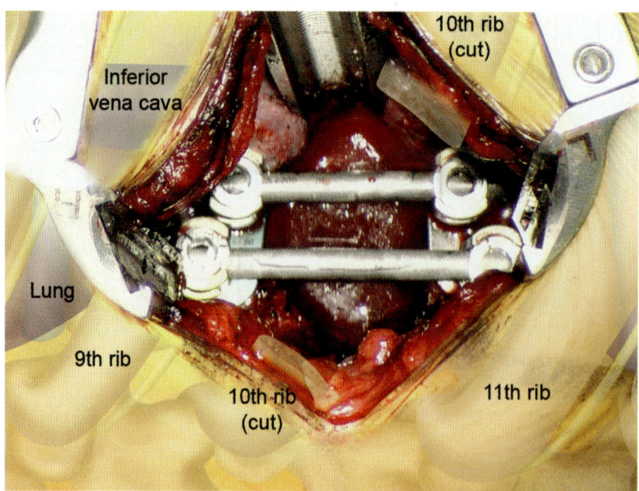

Fig. 6.11: The final rods connecting the two plates are placed to secure the construct between the adjacent levels.

- Step 4
  - Final fixation is achieved with the placement of a dual rod construct (Fig. 6.11).
    - Percutaneous pedicle screws are utilized to supplement the fixation. This is performed in a lateral decubitus position or by placing the patient into a prone position on a Jackson table.

Step 4 Pearls

- A red rubber catheter/chest tube can be placed prior to closure to remove the air from the retropleural space. The red rubber catheter is left in place and clamped.

POSTOPERATIVE CARE (FIGS. 6.12A TO C)

Chest X-Ray

- A plain chest film radiograph is obtained on postoperative day 1 to evaluate for a pleural effusion or pneumothorax. If the chest X-ray is clear, the red rubber catheter can be safely removed and an occlusive dressing is placed.

Complications

- Intercostal neuralgia
- Incidental durotomy
  - A combination of fibrin glue/tissue sealants/fat grafts should be utilized to seal the durotomy. Gentle tamponade of the defect for 10–20 minutes will allow reconstitution of the arachnoid. Persistent dural leaks in the thoracic retropleural space can be challenging to manage after surgery.
- Atelectasis
- Pneumothorax
  - If a red rubber catheter was left in place after surgery, it should be placed to suction. Serial chest X-rays should be done.
  - A chest tube is necessary in cases of a massive pneumothorax or in cases where a pleural effusion is also present.
- Pneumonia

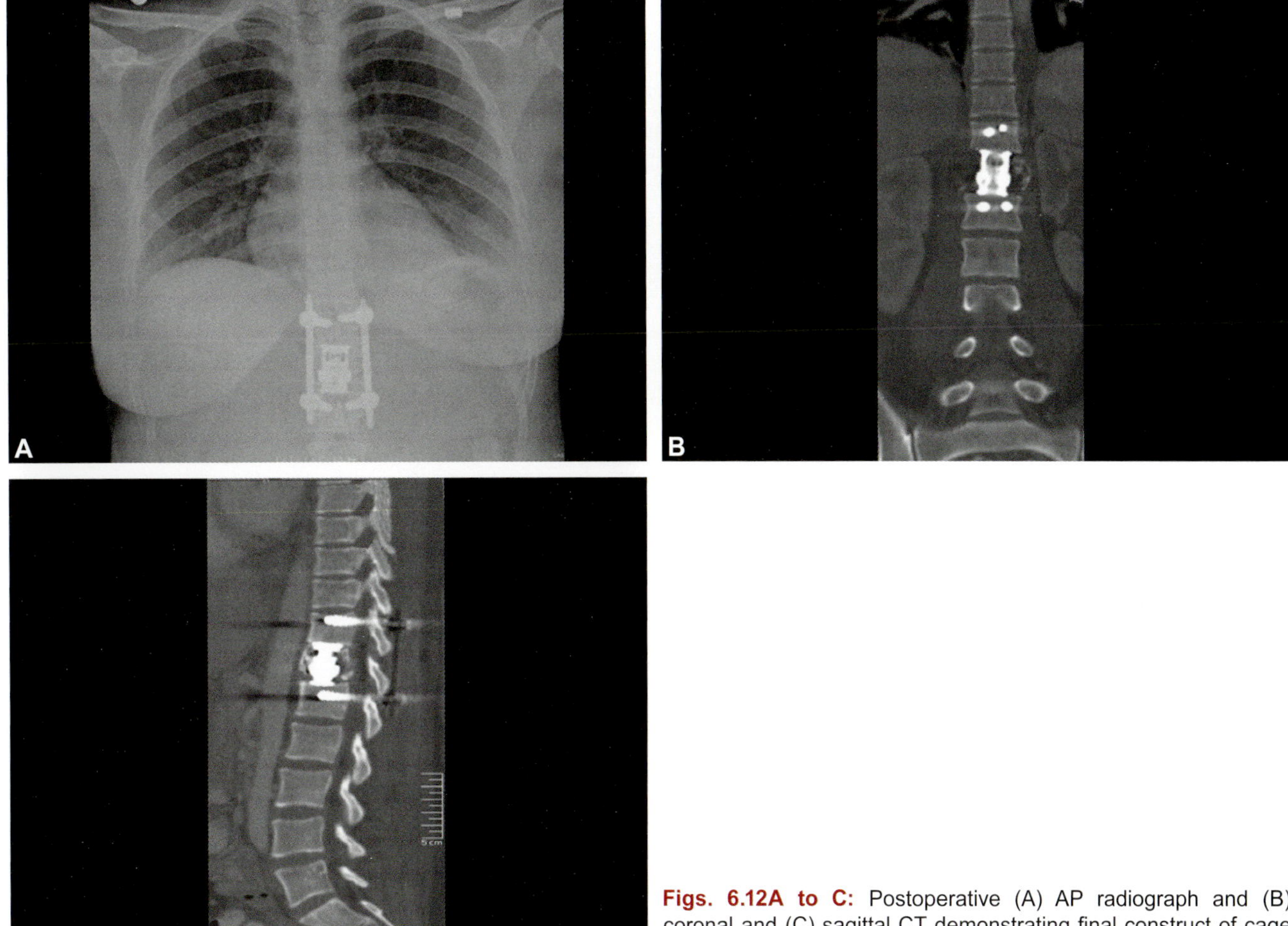

Figs. 6.12A to C: Postoperative (A) AP radiograph and (B) coronal and (C) sagittal CT demonstrating final construct of cage after T12 corpectomy.

EXPECTED AND ADVERSE OUTCOMES

Minimally invasive retropleural thoracic exposures are associated with a shorter procedural time, reduced blood loss, and decreased hospitalization. The rate of complications including intercostal neuralgia, urinary retention, durotomy, lower extremity weakness, atelectasis, pleural effusion, pneumonia, and posterior hardware infection is significantly lower than a traditional open approach.[1,2]

REFERENCES

1. Uribe JS, Smith WD, Pimenta L, et al. Minimally invasive lateral approach for symptomatic thoracic disc herniation: initial multicenter clinical experience. J Neurosurg Spine. 2012;16:264-79.
2. Smith WD, Dakwar E, Le TV, et al. Minimally invasive surgery for traumatic spinal pathologies—a mini-open, lateral approach in the thoracic and lumbar spine. Spine. 2010;35:S338-46.

REFERENCE SUMMARY

1. Uribe JS, Smith WD, Pimenta L, et al. Minimally invasive lateral approach for symptomatic thoracic disc herniation: initial multicenter clinical experience. Journal of Neurosurgery Spine 2012;16:264-79.
   Summary: A multicenter study of 60 patients who underwent a mini-open lateral approach for symptomatic thoracic herniated discs. The authors reported a reduced blood loss, procedural time, hospitalization, and post-operative complications when compared with the traditional open approach.
2. Smith WD, Dakwar E, Le TV, et al. Minimally invasive surgery for traumatic spinal pathologies—a mini-open, lateral approach in the thoracic and lumbar spine. Spine 2010;35:S338-46.
   Summary: Thirty-eight of the 52 (73%) patients who underwent a minimally invasive retropleural approach for a thoracic spine procedure demonstrated either complete neurological recovery or minimal residual deficits (American Spinal Injury Association E or D).

Chapter

7

Percutaneous Cement Augmentation

Alejandro Marquez-Lara, Daniel K Park

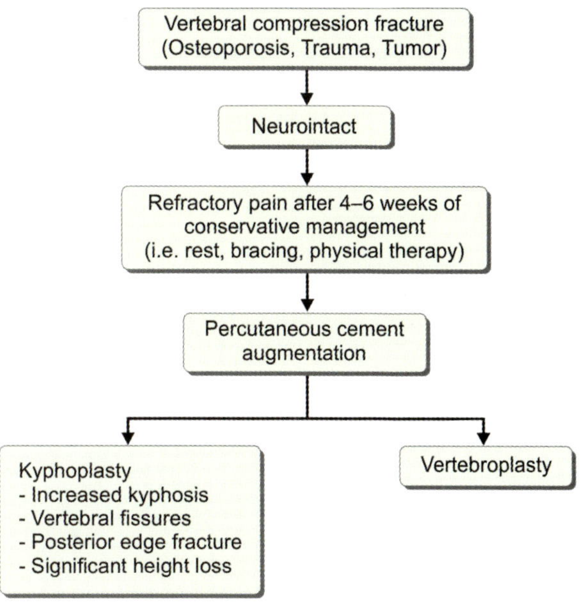

CASE VIGNETTE

An 83-year-old woman with a history of osteoporosis presents to the office with sudden onset thoracic back pain. The patient denies any trauma-related injury. She states that the pain worsens with standing and ambulation but is relieved when lying supine. On examination, the patient demonstrates a slightly kyphotic posture with tenderness to palpation over the T12–L1 spinous processes. There is no evidence of motor or sensory deficit. After 6 weeks of conservative management with physical therapy, pain medication, and bracing the patient continues to have debilitating pain in her back.

DIAGNOSTIC IMAGING

- Plain film radiograph—Anteroposterior (AP) and lateral
  - Plain radiographs in two orthogonal planes enable visualization of the vertebral bodies for evidence of collapse and instability.
    - Plain films also enable assessment of the pedicles to determine if they will be easily identified during the procedure.

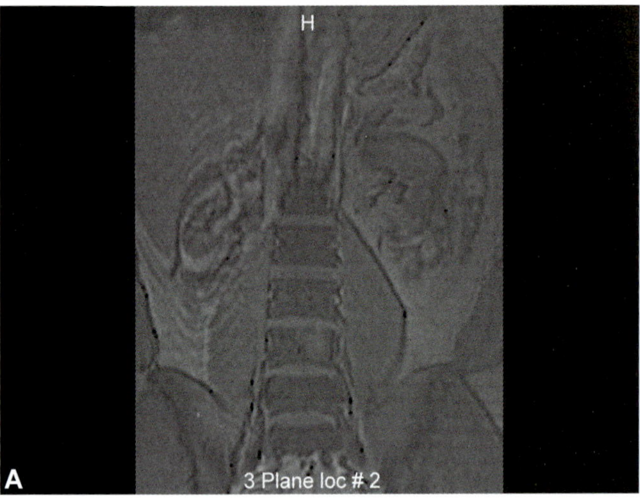

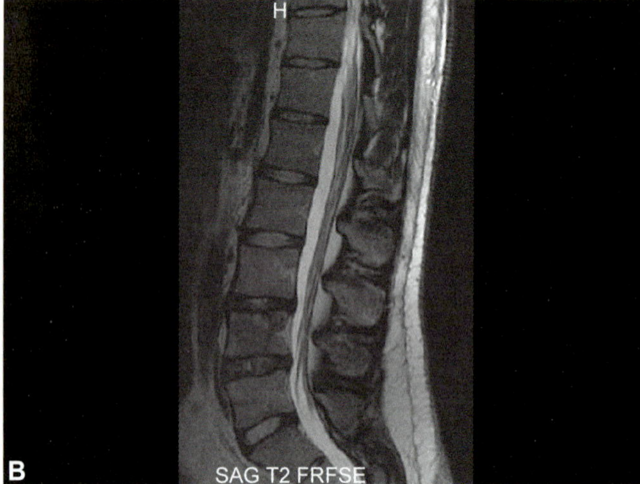

Figs. 7.1A and B: Preoperative coronal (A) and sagittal (B) magnetic resonance imaging demonstrating a nondisplaced compression fracture at L4.

- Magnetic resonance imaging (MRI) (Figs. 7.1A and B)
  - An MRI allows evaluation of the age of the fracture through evidence of bone edema on the T2-weighted images.
  - Often performed to evaluate if the bone fragments are compressing adjacent neural structures.
  - MRI can also assess the degree of structural stability and the competency of the posterior ligamentous complex.
- Computed tomography (CT)
  - A CT scan can characterize the fracture pattern and the integrity of the posterior vertebral body wall.
  - Careful assessment of the vertebral body is essential to determine if the cement will be contained within the vertebral body.
  - A CT scan is also helpful to evaluate suspected lytic lesions.

SURGICAL INDICATIONS

Vertebral Compression Fractures with Refractory or Debilitating Pain

- Trauma
  - Stable
  - Unstable—Cement augmentation may be utilized as an adjuvant during posterior stabilization.
- Pathologic fractures
  - Oncologic
    - Primary
    - Metastatic
  - Osteoporotic

Instrumentation

- Radiolucent table
- Intraoperative fluoroscopy
  - 1 or 2 C-arms (AP and lateral)

Absolute Contraindications

- Bone cement allergy
- Asymptomatic fractures
- Neurological symptoms associated with severe stenosis
- Active infection
- Extension of tumor into the spinal canal
- Chronic fractures
- Uncorrectable coagulopathy

Relative Contraindications

- Burst fracture
- Fractured pedicles
- Vertebra plana
- >3 spinal segments

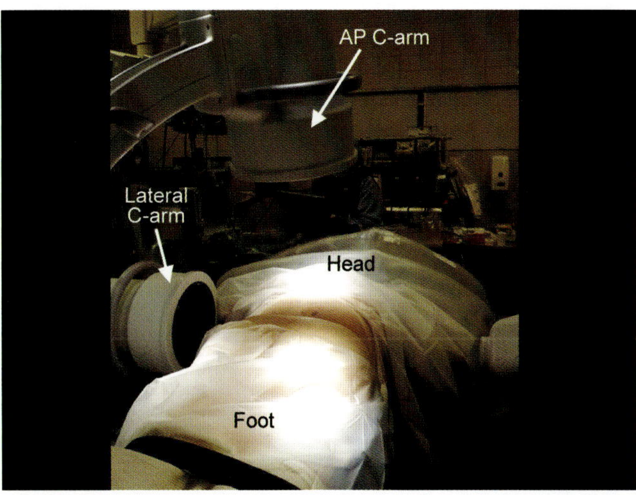

Fig. 7.2: The patient is placed prone and two C-arms are positioned to allow for biplanar fluoroscopy throughout the procedure.

- Spinal access cannula
- Balloon catheter (kyphoplasty)
- Cement-Polymethylmethacrylate

> **Instrumentation Pearls**
> - A single batch of cement can be utilized for multiple levels. To delay the polymerization process, the cement is stored in a sterile ice water bath.
> - The cement load determines the number of levels that can be treated. In general, no more than three levels are treated in one operation to avoid monomer toxicity.

POSITIONING AND INTRAOPERATIVE SETUP

- The procedure can be performed under monitored anesthesia care or general anesthesia with endotracheal intubation.
- The patient is placed into a prone position on a radiolucent table.
  - Appropriate padding is placed over the bony prominences.
- Fluoroscope placement (Fig. 7.2)
  - The AP fluoroscope is brought in with the image intensifier directly over the target site.
    - If two C-arms are utilized, it is recommended to obtain a true AP image prior to positioning the second fluoroscope in the lateral position.
  - The lateral image fluoroscope can then be brought into the field over or under the patient's trunk with the arc angled toward the patient's head.
  - Confirmation of the pedicle image should be done both in the AP and lateral planes.

SURGICAL ANATOMY

- Relevant anatomy (Figs. 7.3A to G)
  - The medial wall of the thoracic pedicle is thicker than the lateral wall.
  - The thoracic pedicles have a decreasing medial angulation in the transverse plane from T1 (~30°) to T12 (~7°). In the sagittal plane, the pedicles have a 10°–20° cephalad angulation (Figs. 7.3A and C).
  - The lumbar pedicles have an increasing medial angulation in the transverse plane from L1 (5°–10°) to L5 (20°–30°). In the sagittal plane, the lumbar pedicles have a relatively shallow caudal angulation between 2°–10° (Figs. 7.3B and D).

MRI ~ sagittal thoracic model
Sagittal plane angle –
T1 – 10-12°
T2 – 15-22°
T3 – 14-20°
T4 – 13-18°
T5 – 15-20°
T6 – 14-18°
T7 – 12-17°
T8 – 12-17°
T9 – 11-16°
T10 – 11-16°
T11 – 12-14°
T12 – 10-12°
C7
T1
T2
T3
T4
T5
T6
T7
T8
T9
T10
T11
T12
L1
A
MRI ~ sagittal lumbar model
Sagittal plane angle –
L1 – 5-10°
L2 – 5-7°
L3 – 4-5°
L4 – 3-4°
L5 – 2-3°
L1
L2
L3
L4
L5
B
Transverse plane angle — 15–20°
T5
C
Transverse plane angle — 10–15°
T9
D
Transverse plane angle — 5–10°
L1
E
Transverse plane angle — 10–20°
L3
F

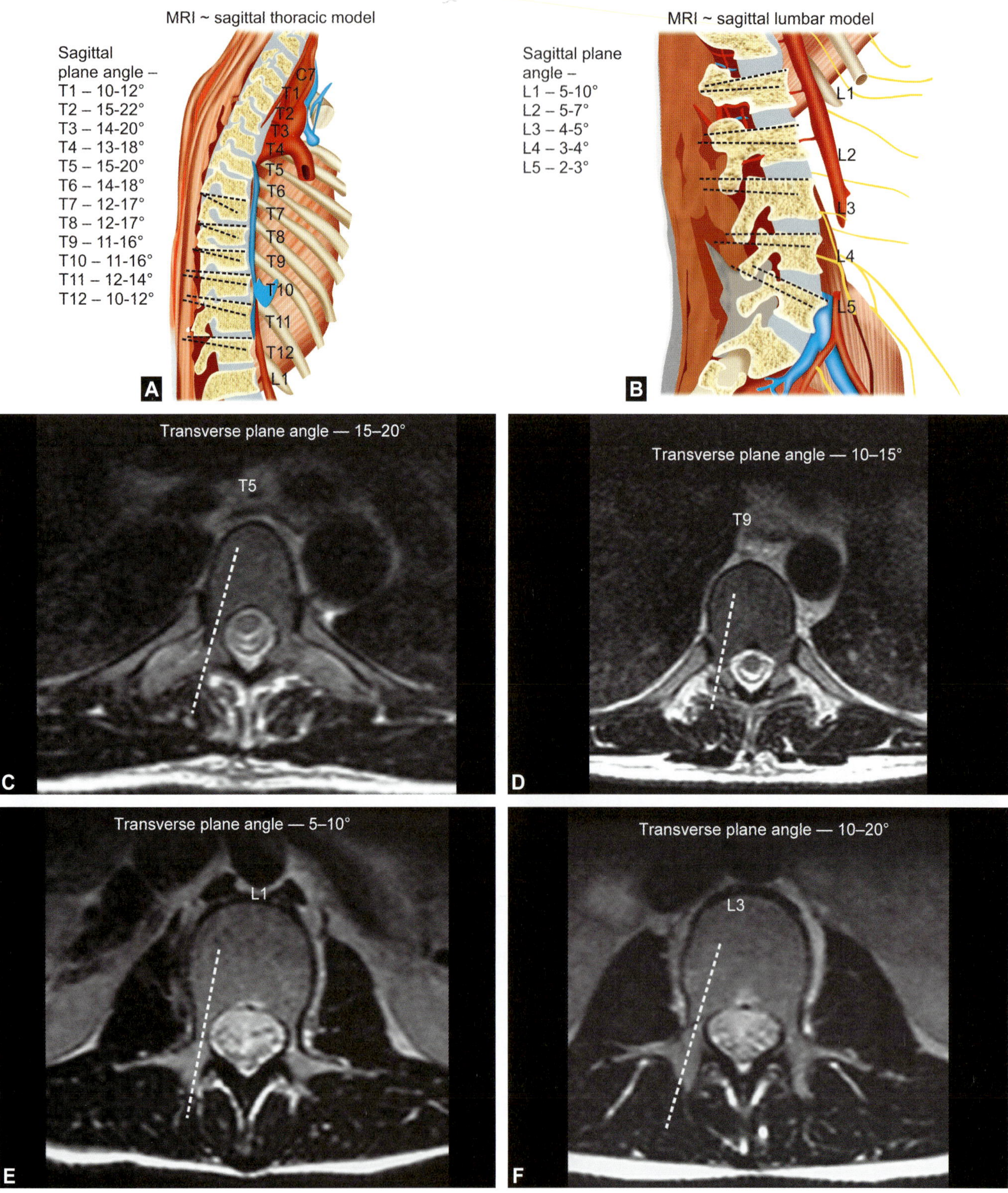

Figs. 7.3A to F

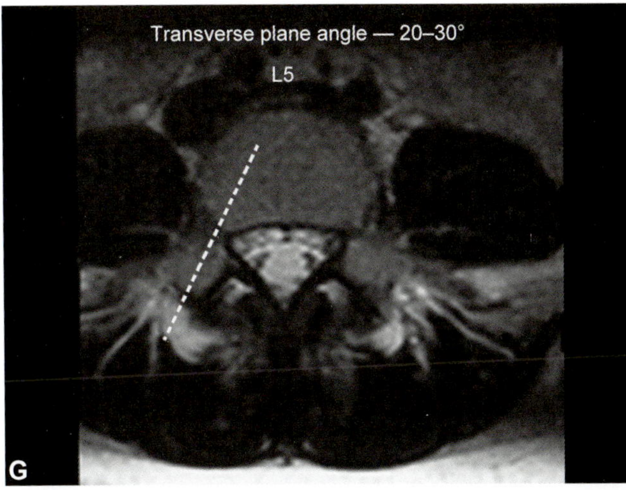

Figs. 7.3A to G: Illustration of a sagittal cut of the thoracic (A) and lumbar (B) spine demonstrating the pedicle angulation in the sagittal plane. Axial computer tomographic scans of different thoracic (C and D) and lumbar (E–G) vertebrae depicting the pedicle orientation in the transverse plane.

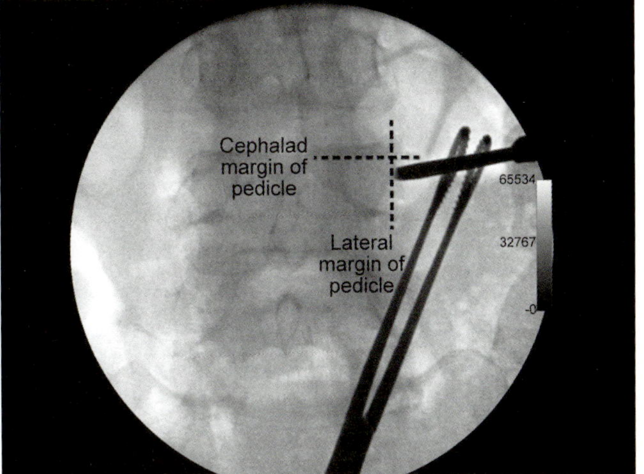

Fig. 7.4: An anteroposterior intraoperative fluoroscopy depicting the intersection of the cephalad and lateral margins of the pedicle, which can help guide the site for the skin incision.

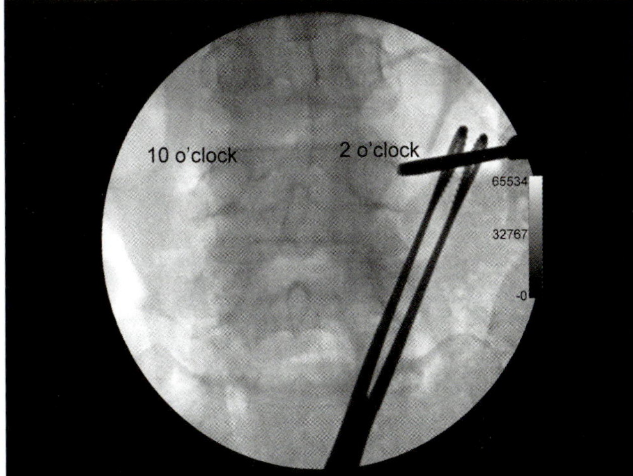

Fig. 7.5: An anteroposterior radiograph demonstrating the correct starting point for the spinal access needle.

PROCEDURE-SPECIFIC STEPS

- Step 1
  - After identifying the level of interest, a 5–10 mm longitudinal stab incision is made 10 mm lateral to the lateral pedicle wall on the radiograph.
    - The intersection of the cephalad and lateral margin of the pedicle in the AP view may be utilized as a guide for the skin incision (Fig. 7.4).
  - A cannulated spinal access needle is angled medially and placed at the intersection of the lateral border of the superior facet and a bisecting line of the transverse process (Fig. 7.5).
    - The starting position for the cannula should be on the superior-lateral corner of the pedicle (2 o'clock on the right side and 10 o'clock on the left side).
    - This position places the cannula the farthest from the exiting nerve root (directly underneath the pedicle).

Procedure Pearls

- With a vertebroplasty, all of the cannulas are inserted first and then each site is injected sequentially.
- With a kyphoplasty, the first site is cannulated, the balloon is deployed, and the cement injected.

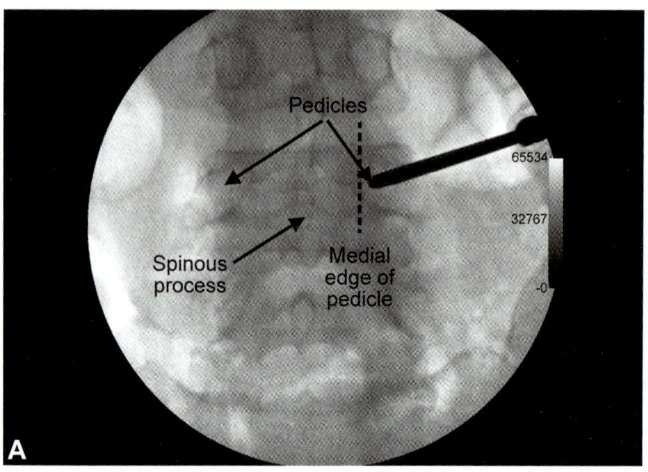

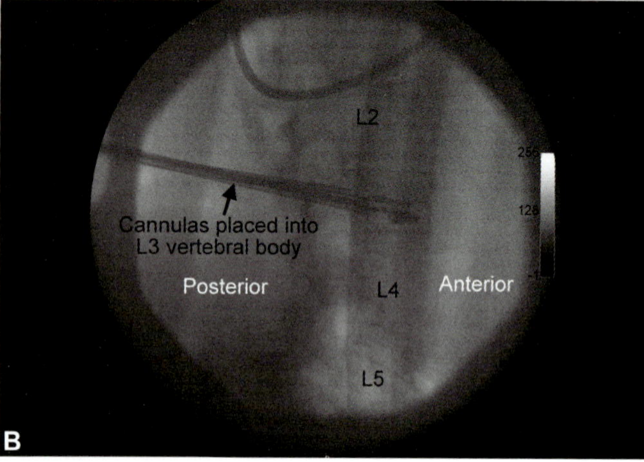

Figs. 7.6A and B: Anteroposterior (A) and lateral (B) intraoperative fluoroscopy demonstrating the cannulated access needle passed the posterior wall of the vertebral body while respecting the medial edge of the pedicle.

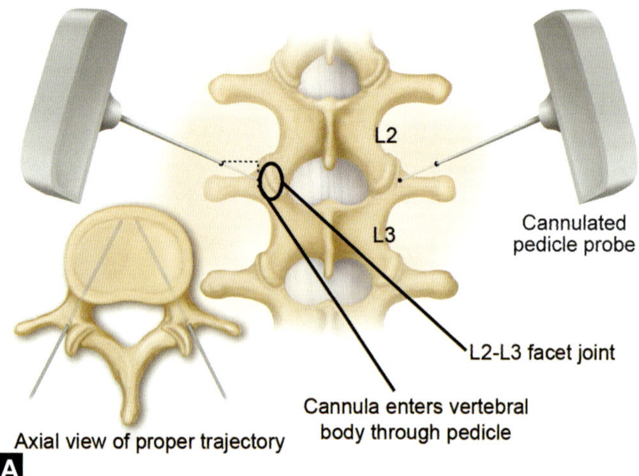

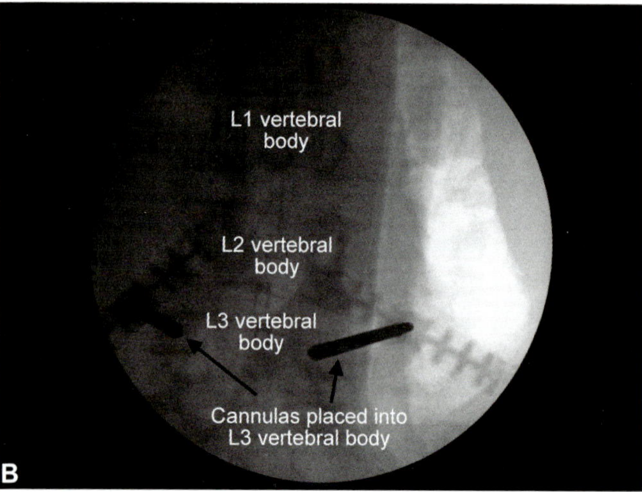

Figs. 7.7A and B: Intraoperative picture (A) and anteroposterior radiograph (B) demonstrating the correct position for bilateral cannulated access needles.

- Step 2
  - The cannula is advanced with a gentle twisting motion or with a mallet under direct AP and lateral fluoroscopy in increments of 5 mm.
  - Care should be taken to avoid crossing the medial wall of the pedicle on the AP view, until the tip of the cannula crosses the line of the posterior vertebral body on the lateral image (Figs. 7.6A and B).
    - If the tip of the cannula crosses the medial wall of the pedicle prior to reaching the line of the posterior vertebral body (15–20 mm) the trajectory should be re-evaluated as a medial wall breech is likely.
  - The process is then repeated on the contralateral pedicle and any of the other levels involved (Figs. 7.7A and B).
- Step 3
  - For a kyphoplasty, once the position of the cannula is confirmed, the balloon taps are advanced into the anterior portion of the vertebral body and inflated (Figs. 7.8A and B).

Procedure Pearls

- If one C-arm to stay consistent is utilized, the cannula can be advanced 15–20 mm so long as the tip is lateral to the medial pedicle wall. A lateral image is then obtained to ensure the cannula tip is anterior to the posterior margin of the vertebral body.

Procedure Pearls

- Unilateral cannulation can be performed if the cannula tip is close to the midline of the vertebral body.

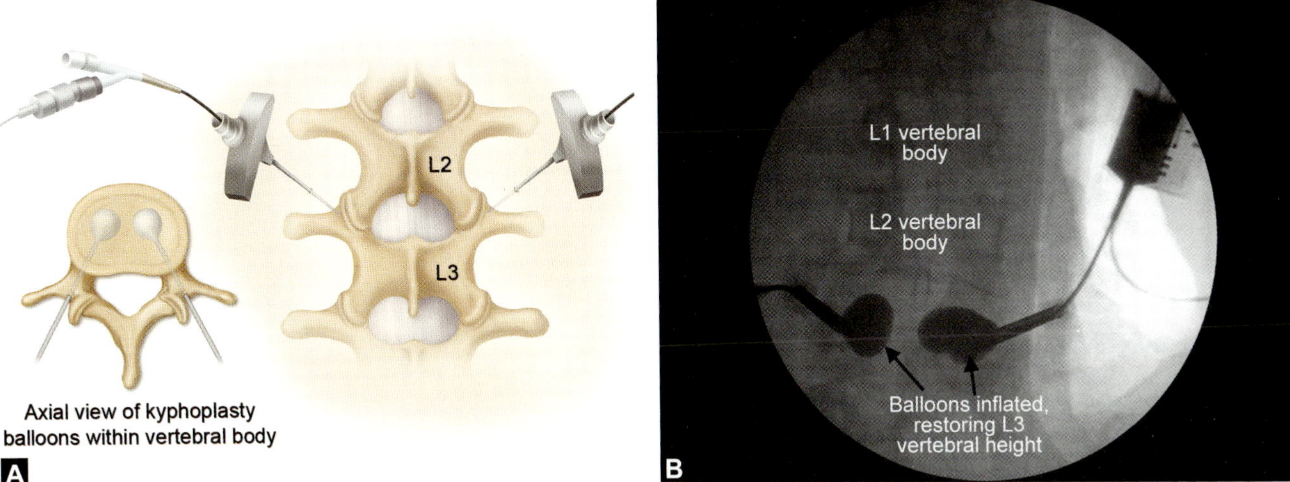

Figs. 7.8A and B: Intraoperative picture (A) and anteroposterior radiograph (B) demonstrating the inflation of kyphoplasty balloons within the vertebral body.

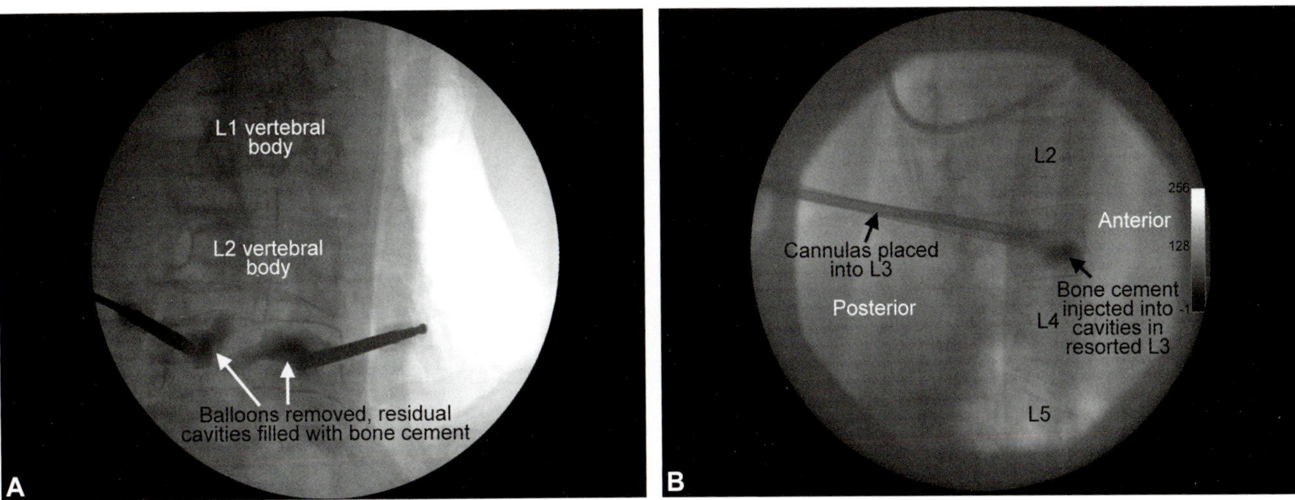

Figs. 7.9A and B: Anteroposterior (A) and lateral (B) intraoperative fluoroscopy demonstrating bone cement being injected into the affected vertebral body.

- Making sure that the balloons are in the anterior portion of the vertebral body, prevents retropulsion of bone into the vertebral canal when the balloons are inflated.

- Step 4
  - The cement is then sequentially added to the vertebral body under AP and lateral fluoroscopic guidance (Figs. 7.9A and B).
    - If the borders of the vertebral bodies are violated or cement extravasation is noted the procedure should be terminated.
    - Cement should be avoided in the posterior aspect of the vertebral body.
  - At the end of the procedure, the cement filling should approach the midline in the AP view (Figs. 7.10A and B).

Procedure Pearls

- In general, the volume of cement injected should be greater than the volume of the inflated balloon. This will prevent iatrogenic vertebral body collapse.
- An "eggshell" technique can be utilized to help maintain the fracture reduction. After the initial deployment of the balloon tamp, a small amount of cement (4-5 mL) is injected in the cavity. The balloon tamp is reinserted and gently expanded to create a thin shell of cement to hold the reduction.

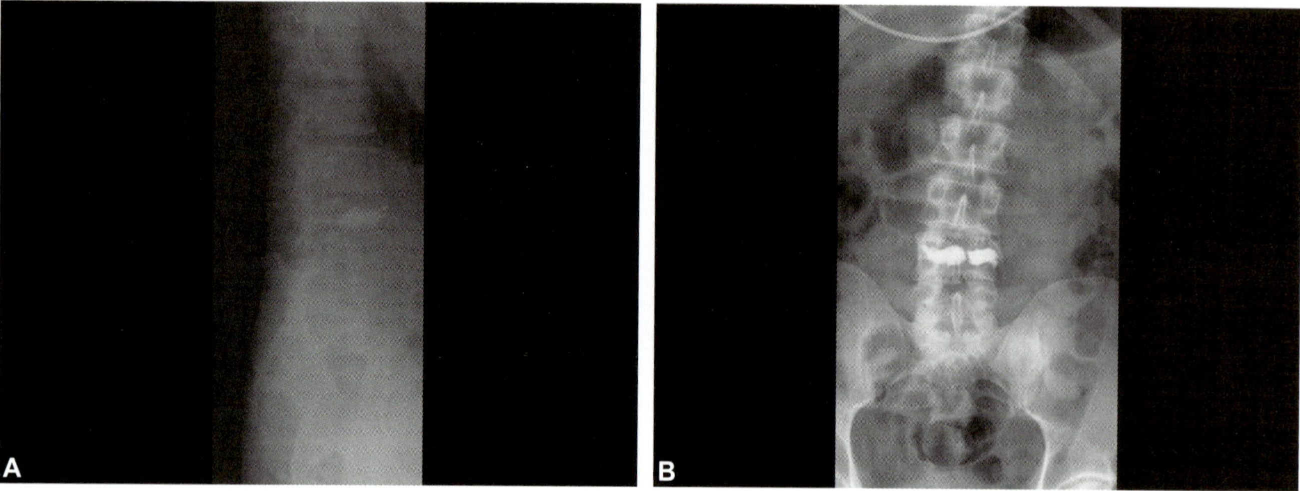

Figs. 7.10A and B: Anteroposterior (A) and lateral (B) postoperative radiograph after L4 vertebral body cement augmentation.

COMPLICATIONS

- Cement extravasation (13–52%)—Most are asymptomatic.
  - Cement extravasation into the neuroforamen or spinal canal can result in radicular or myelopathic symptoms.
  - Cement leakage into the neighboring venous system may lead to a cement pulmonary embolism. However, most of these are asymptomatic and routine chest X-ray or CT scans are not recommended.
- Adjacent level compression fractures.
  - Studies have demonstrated a 38% incidence of adjacent level compression fractures after cement augmentation. However, the principal risk factor remains a low bone density T-score and the number of vertebral fractures.[1]

EXPECTED AND ADVERSE OUTCOMES

- Cement leakage occurs in 52% of vertebroplasties and 13% of kyphoplasties.[1,2] However, very few are symptomatic (0–0.8%) (Figs. 7.11A and B). The reduced leakage rate observed after kyphoplasty procedures may be related to the injection of high-viscosity cement at a low pressure.
- Patients with refractory pain from osteoporotic vertebral compression fractures (OVCF) who are treated with either a kyphoplasty or vertebroplasty may demonstrate a higher long-term survival rate when compared with those who are treated conservatively.[3]
- Kyphoplasty procedures are safe and effective minimally invasive interventions for the management of OVCF. A randomized control trial demonstrated a significant benefit of kyphoplasty over conservative treatment at 1 month; however, effectiveness decreased at 12 months.[4]
- There is conflicting evidence in the literature regarding the benefits of vertebroplasty for the treatment of OVCF.[1,5] However, two randomized double-blinded placebo-controlled trials have demonstrated no treatment benefit of vertebroplasty over a sham procedure.[6,7]

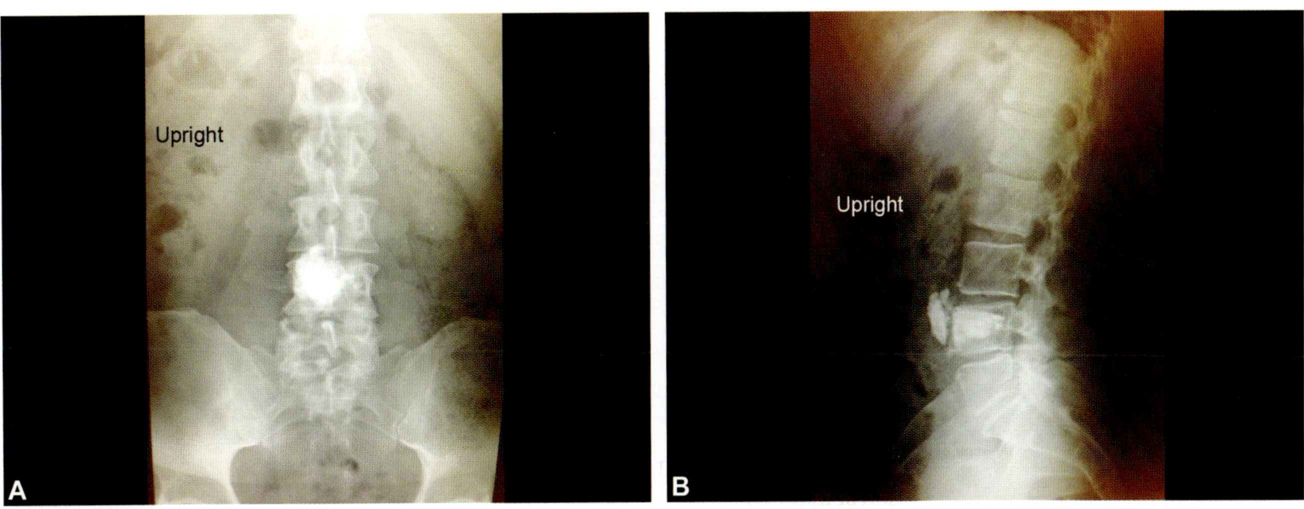

Figs. 7.11A and B: Anteroposterior (A) and lateral (B) postoperative radiograph demonstrating asymptomatic anterior leak due to uncontained cement.

- The American Academy of Orthopedic Surgeons analyzed the published literature regarding cement bone augmentation. The organization recommended against vertebroplasty while giving kyphoplasty a "weak recommendation" for the treatment of OVCF.

REFERENCES

1. Asenjo JF, Rossel F. Vertebroplasty and kyphoplasty: new evidence adds heat to the debate. Curr Opin Anaesthesiol. 2012;25:577-83.
2. Lee MJ, Dumonski M, Cahill P, et al. Percutaneous treatment of vertebral compression fractures—a meta-analysis of complications. Spine. 2009;34: 1228-32.
3. Gerling MC, Eubanks JD, Patel R, et al. Cement augmentation of refractory osteoporotic vertebral compression fractures: survivorship analysis. Spine (Phila Pa 1976). 2011;36:E1266-9.
4. Wardlaw D, Cummings SR, Van Meirhaeghe J, et al. Efficacy and safety of balloon kyphoplasty compared with non-surgical care for vertebral compression fracture (FREE): a randomised controlled trial. Lancet. 2009; 373:1016-24.
5. Klazen CA, Lohle PN, de Vries J, et al. Vertebroplasty versus conservative treatment in acute osteoporotic vertebral compression fractures (Vertos II): an open-label randomised trial. Lancet. 2010;376:1085-92.
6. Buchbinder R, Osborne RH, Ebeling PR, Wark JD. A randomized trial of vertebroplasty for painful osteoporotic vertebral fractures. N Engl J Med. 2009;361:557-68.
7. Kallmes DF, Comstock BA, Heagerty PJ, et al. A randomized trial of vertebroplasty for osteoporotic spinal fractures. N Engl J Med. 2009;361: 569-79.

REFERENCE SUMMARY

1. Asenjo JF, Rossel F. Vertebroplasty and kyphoplasty: new evidence adds heat to the debate. Current Opinion in Anaesthesiology. 2012;25:577-83.

Summary: The controversial evidence surrounding the benefits of cement bone augmentation is addressed through a literature review of well-designed prospective clinical trials and meta-analyses. The authors report that cement augmentation techniques are associated with better and faster pain relief and improved functional outcomes when compared with conservative management.

2. Lee MJ, Dumonski M, Cahill P, et al. Percutaneous treatment of vertebral compression fractures—a meta-analysis of complications. Spine. 2009;34: 1228-32.
   Summary: A meta-analysis comparing complication rates from vertebroplasty (VP) and kyphoplasty (KP). The authors analyzed 121 studies and reported that VP was found to have a significantly increased rate of procedure-related complications and cement leakage (symptomatic and asymptomatic).
3. Gerling MC, Eubanks JD, Patel R, et al. Cement augmentation of refractory osteoporotic vertebral compression fractures: survivorship analysis. Spine. (Phila Pa 1976) 2011;36:E1266-9.
   Summary: A literature review on long-term patient survival after an OVCF treated with either cement augmentation or traditional conservative management. The authors report a significant survival advantage after cement augmentation compared with controls.
4. Wardlaw D, Cummings SR, Van Meirhaeghe J, et al. Efficacy and safety of balloon kyphoplasty compared with non-surgical care for vertebral compression fracture (FREE): a randomised controlled trial. Lancet 2009;373:1016-1024.
   Summary: A randomized controlled trial comparing balloon kyphoplasty versus conservative treatment for patients with acute vertebral fractures. Although kyphoplasty demonstrated better outcomes when compared with conservative treatment, for most outcome measures, the differences between groups were diminished at 12 months.
5. Klazen CA, Lohle PN, de Vries J, et al. Vertebroplasty versus conservative treatment in acute osteoporotic vertebral compression fractures (Vertos II): an open-label randomised trial. Lancet 2010;376:1085-92.
   Summary: A randomized controlled trial comparing the improvement in clinical outcomes and quality of life scores in patients undergoing vertebroplasty versus conservative treatment for vertebral compression fractures. The authors concluded that vertebroplasty is an effective and safe procedure to achieve better immediate and sustained (1 year) pain relief than conservative treatment.
6. Buchbinder R, Osborne RH, Ebeling PR, Wark JD. A randomized trial of vertebroplasty for painful osteoporotic vertebral fractures. N Engl J Med. 2009;361:557-68.
   Summary: A multicenter, double-blind, placebo-controlled trial of 78 patients with one or two painful osteoporotic vertebral fractures who were randomized to undergo a vertebroplasty or a Sham procedure. The authors reported no significant benefits associated with a vertebroplasty over a Sham procedure at 1 week or at 1, 3, or 6 months after intervention.
7. Kallmes DF, Comstock BA, Heagerty PJ, et al. A randomized trial of vertebroplasty for osteoporotic spinal fractures. N Engl J Med. 2009;361:569-79.
   Summary: A multicenter, double-blinded, placebo-controlled trial of 131 patients with one to three painful OVCF who were randomized to either a vertebroplasty or Sham procedure. The authors reported a similar improvement between the two study cohorts.

Chapter

8

Minimally Invasive Lumbar Discectomy

Sreeharsha V Nandyala, Gabriel Duhancioglu, Daniel D Bohl, Kern Singh

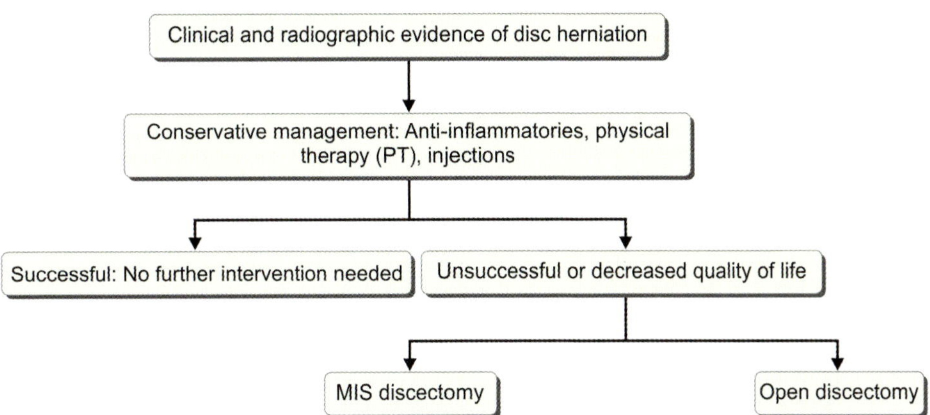

CASE VIGNETTE

A 48-year-old woman presents to the office with worsening back pain that radiates to her left lower extremity. On examination, the patient demonstrates radicular symptoms consistent with an S1 nerve root impingement. She demonstrates weakness in her left gastrocnemius as well as a diminished Achilles tendon reflex.

DIAGNOSTIC IMAGING

- Plain film radiograph—Anteroposterior (AP) and lateral
  - Helps evaluate for osseous abnormalities in the lumbar spine that may interfere with an adequate exposure (i.e. rudimentary sacral disc, spina bifida oculta).
  - Can also evaluate for transitional vertebrae (lumbarized sacrum)
- Magnetic resonance imaging (Figs. 8.1A and B)
  - Provides a detailed assessment of the disc herniation and its anatomic location, which will help guide intraoperative localization

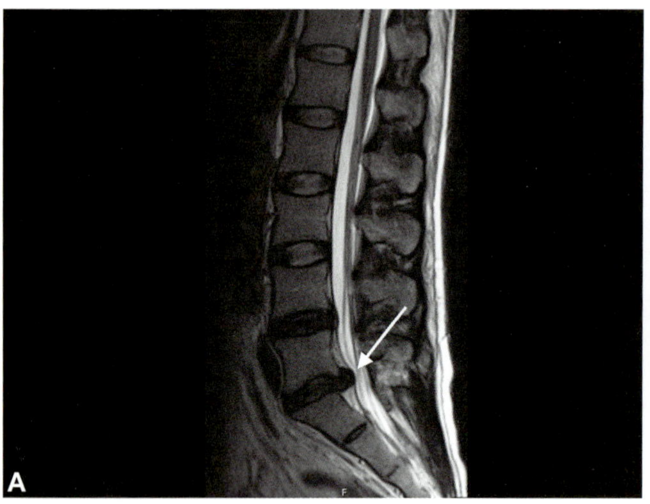

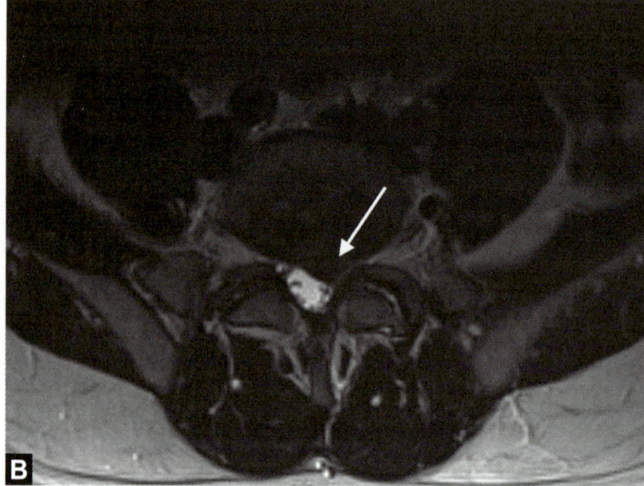

Figs. 8.1A and B: Preoperative (A) sagittal and (B) axial magnetic resonance image demonstrating a left posterolateral herniated nucleus pulposus.

SURGICAL INDICATIONS

- Herniated nucleus pulposus (HNP) in the lumbar spine
  - Radiculopathy
  - Motor weakness
  - Persistent pain
  - Failed conservative management

Indication Pearls

- Far lateral disc herniation affects the exiting nerve root as it exits the neuroforamen at the level of the disc space. In this situation, a far lateral discectomy is recommended.

INSTRUMENTATION

- Jackson table
- Intraoperative fluoroscopy
- Surgical microscope or magnifying loupes
- Sequential dilators
- Tubular retractor
- Microscopic instrumentation
  - Rongeurs
  - Curettes
  - Burrs
- Electrocautery

Instrumentation Pearls

- A smaller diameter retractor may improve intraoperative visualization in situations of a congenitally narrowed spinal canal by allowing placement of the tube medial to the facet joint.

POSITIONING AND INTRAOPERATIVE SETUP

- The patient is placed into a prone position on a Jackson table (Fig. 8.2).
  - The abdomen is allowed to hang freely to reduce the intra-abdominal pressure and prevent secondary venous congestion.
- The arms are abducted and the elbows are flexed at 90°.
  - Appropriate padding is placed over the bony prominences (elbows, patella).
- A chest roll is placed to maximize the lumbar lordosis.
- The surgeon should be positioned on the side of the pathology while the fluoroscope, monitor, and microscope are placed on the contralateral side.

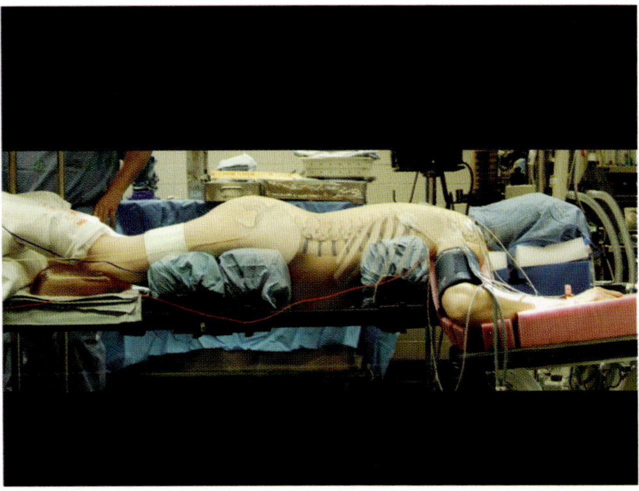

Fig. 8.2: The patient laying prone on a Jackson table with appropriate padding for the chest, hips, thighs, knees, and arms.

LUMBAR DISCECTOMY

Surgical Anatomy and Exposure

Relevant Anatomy

- Identification of the pedicle is key for intraoperative localization of the disc space and the nerve root.
  - The inferolateral corner of the interlaminar space is a reliable landmark for localizing the pedicle. Detachment of the ligamentum flavum at this landmark exposes the medial wall of the pedicle.
    - The disc space is 5–10 mm above the pedicle, and the traversing nerve root is just medial to the medial edge of the pedicle.

Surgical

- The appropriate level is identified under fluoroscopic guidance.
- A 1–2-cm longitudinal skin incision is made 1.5 cm lateral to the midline on the side of the pathology. A fasciotomy that is the same length as the skin incision is also performed.
- A starting dilator is introduced to localize the appropriate docking position.
  - On the AP fluoroscopic view, the docking site should be on the inferior portion of the superior lamina, just lateral to the interspinous space.
  - A lateral view alone can also be utilized with the initial dilator sweeping across the superior lamina (tactile feedback) while the C-arm localizes the level of the affected disc space.
- Once the dilator is at the appropriate site, sequential dilation is performed followed by placement of the tubular retractor. The retractor is then secured to the flexible table retractor arm.
- Any remaining overlying muscle and soft tissue is removed with bipolar electrocautery to adequately visualize the anatomic structures.

Exposure Pearls

- Accurate placement of the tubular retractor on both the AP and lateral views will ensure adequate access to the interlaminar space and the intervertebral disc.
- Care must be taken to prevent the retractor from moving once it is in the correct position to avoid distortion of the surgical site.

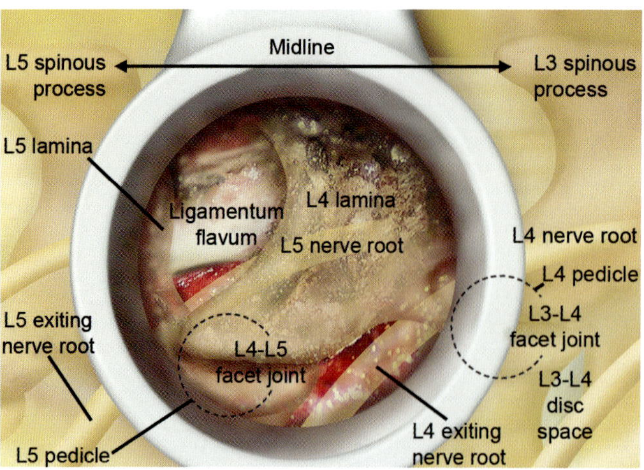

Fig. 8.3: Visualization of the nerve root and disc space after removing the ligamentum flavum, the inferior portion of the superior lamina (L4), and medial aspect of the facet complex.

PROCEDURE-SPECIFIC STEPS—LUMBAR DISCECTOMY

- Step 1
  - The inferior portion of the superior lamina, interlaminar space, and the facet joint are identified (Fig. 8.3).
  - A pituitary rongeur is utilized to remove the soft tissue overlying the ligamentum flavum.
- Step 2
  - Once adequate exposure is obtained, a high-speed burr is utilized to remove the inferior portion of the superior lamina (Figs. 8.4A to C).
    - The laminotomy can extend cephalad until the insertion of the ligamentum flavum.
  - The ligamentum flavum can then be detached with a Kerrison rongeur, thus exposing the dural sac.
  - A partial facetectomy is also performed with the high-speed burr, allowing adequate access to the disc space.
- Step 3
  - The traversing nerve root is gently retracted medially, and any vessels overlying the disc are coagulated with bipolar electrocautery.
  - If necessary, an annulotomy is then performed with a knife.
- Step 4
  - A pituitary rongeur is then utilized to extract any loose fragments of nucleus pulposus.
  - Discectomy continues until there is adequate decompression of the exiting nerve root in the affected foramen.
    - Excursion distance of the nerve (>1 cm) can be utilized as an effective method of determining the adequacy of the discectomy (in addition to direct visualization).

Step 2 Pearls

- Identification of the pars can help determine the lateral extent of the decompression. Greater than 9 mm of pars should be preserved in most situations.

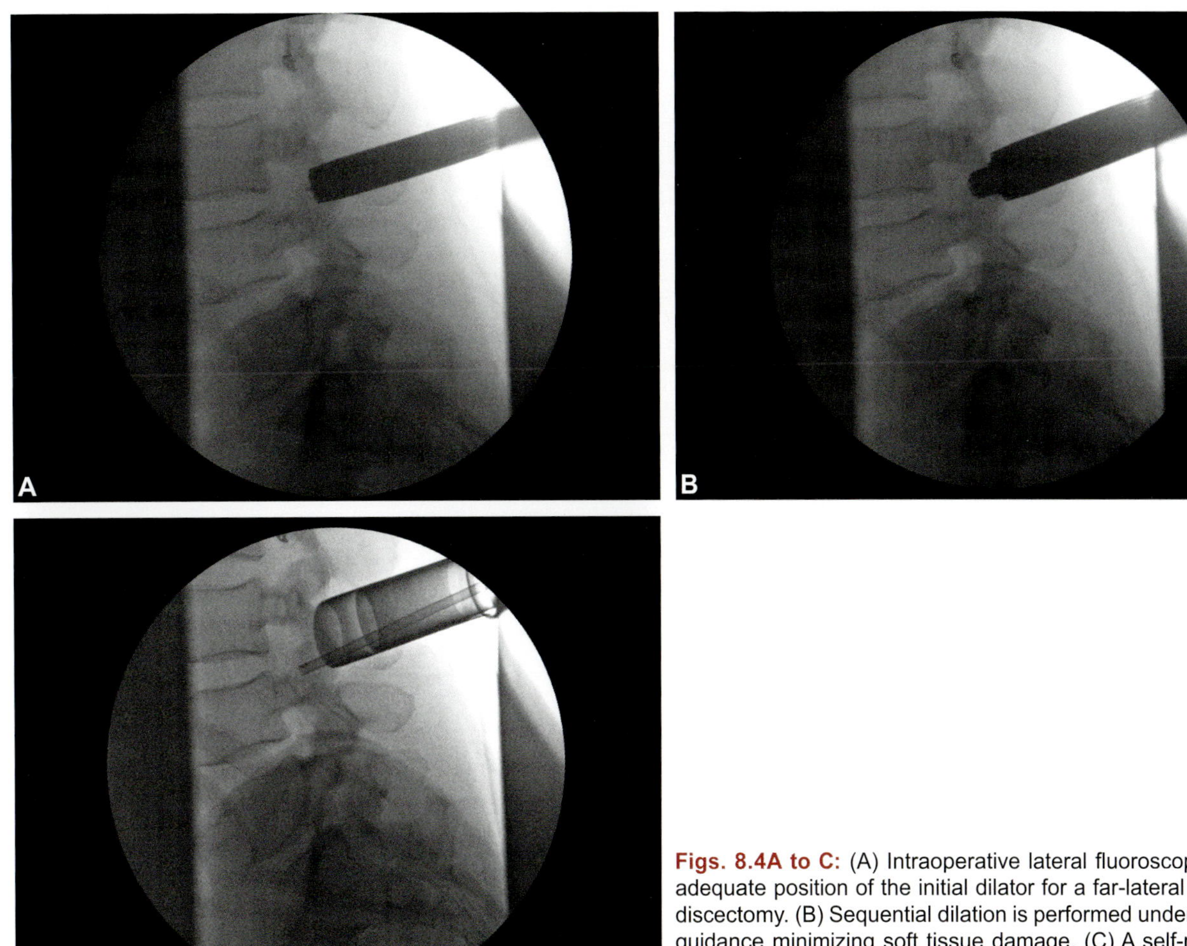

Figs. 8.4A to C: (A) Intraoperative lateral fluoroscopy confirming adequate position of the initial dilator for a far-lateral L3-L4 microdiscectomy. (B) Sequential dilation is performed under fluoroscopic guidance minimizing soft tissue damage. (C) A self-retaining retractor is placed and secured in its final position creating a surgical channel.

FAR-LATERAL LUMBAR DISCECTOMY

Surgical Anatomy and Exposure

Relevant Anatomy

- The dorsal covering of the foraminal zone varies depending upon the lumbar level. At L5, the lateral border of the pars overhangs the foraminal zone. At L4 and above, the lateral border of the pars becomes progressively more medial such that the dorsal covering of the foraminal zone in the proximal levels (L2–L1) is the intertransverse membrane and not the pars.
- The accessory process from the inferior medial edge of the transverse process determines the lateral border of the superior pedicle.
- The exiting nerve roots leave the spinal canal just below the superior pedicle. The disc herniation often displaces the nerve root in a cephalad and lateral direction, pushing the exiting nerve root toward the cephalad pedicle.

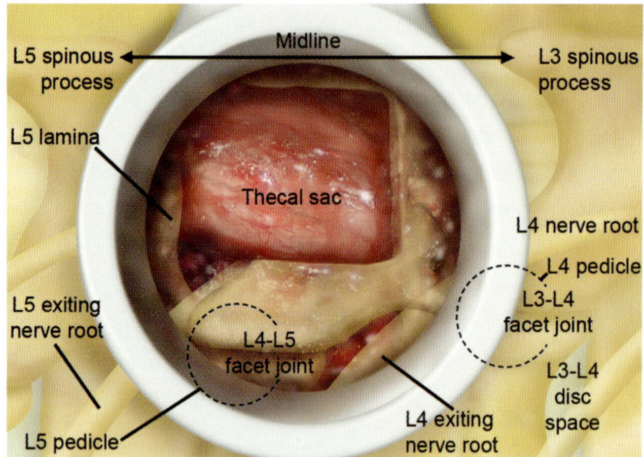

Fig. 8.5: Anatomic landmarks identified through the surgical working channel of a self-retaining retractor.

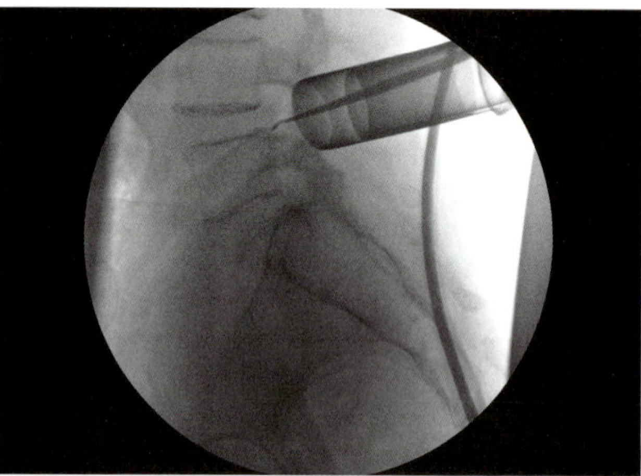

Fig. 8.6: A lateral intraoperative fluoroscopy demonstrating a tubular retractor placed at the appropriate spinal level.

Surgical Exposure

- The appropriate level is identified under AP fluoroscopic guidance (Fig. 8.5).
- A 1–2-cm longitudinal skin incision is made lateral to the pars interarticularis. The trajectory is very similar to that of a pedicle screw for a caudal pedicle.
- A starting dilator is introduced to localize the appropriate docking position.
  - On the AP fluoroscopic view, the docking site should be on the lateral aspect of the pars interarticularis and facet joint and the superior portion of the inferior transverse process.
- Once the dilator is at the appropriate site, sequential dilation is performed followed by placement of the tubular retractor. The retractor is then secured to the flexible table retractor arm (Fig. 8.6).
- Any remaining overlying muscle and soft tissue is removed with bipolar electrocautery to adequately visualize the anatomic structures.

PROCEDURE-SPECIFIC STEPS—FAR-LATERAL LUMBAR DISCECTOMY

- Step 1
  - The lateral aspect of the pars interarticularis, facet joint, and superior border of the inferior transverse process are identified (Fig. 8.7).
    - If L5–S1 is affected, a partial resection of the S1 superior articular process, the caudal part of the L5 transverse process, and the cranial part of the sacral ala may need to be resected with a high-speed burr.
- Step 2
  - The intertransverse membrane is identified and detached from the inferior transverse process with a curved curette and bipolar cautery (Fig. 8.8).
  - If necessary, a small portion of the lateral aspect of the pars interarticularis is resected with a high-speed burr to adequately expose the nerve root.

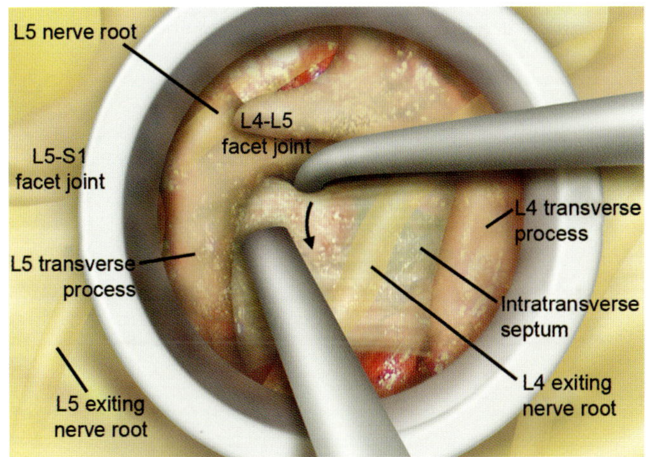

Fig. 8.7: Intraoperative view of the surgical working channel depicting the anatomic landmarks for a far-lateral discectomy.

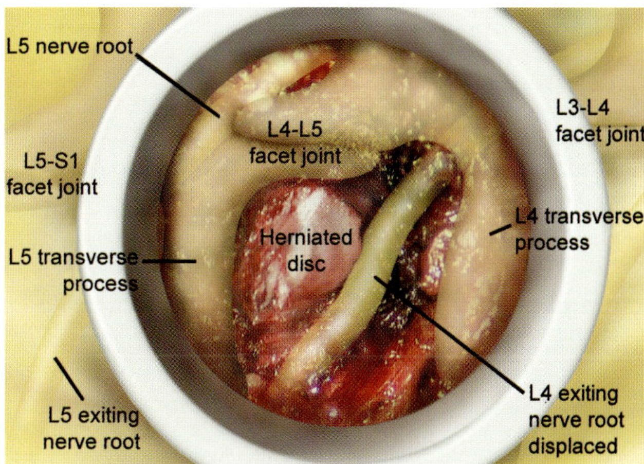

Fig. 8.8: Anatomic structures are better visualized after removing the intertransverse septum.

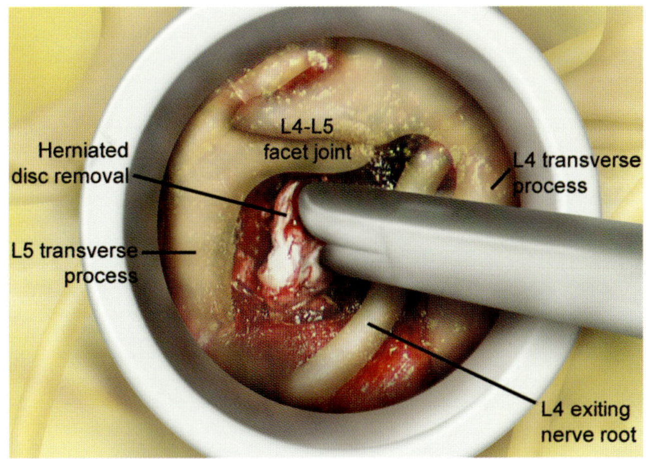

Fig. 8.9: Visualization of a herniated disc compressing and displacing the L4–L5 nerve root.

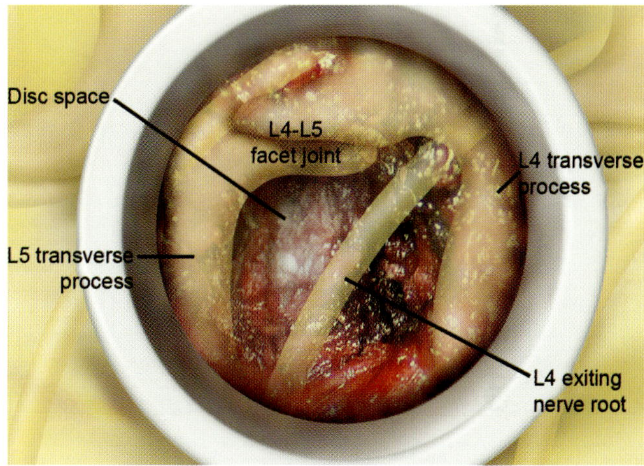

Fig. 8.10: Visualization of the decompressed nerve root following removal of the herniated disc material.

- Step 3
  - The exiting nerve root, which is typically displaced dorsal and lateral to the disc herniation, is then identified (Fig. 8.9).
- Step 4
  - The nerve root is gently retracted superiorly and the disc fragments are removed with a pituitary rongeur (Fig. 8.10).
  - If necessary, after clearly identifying the nerve–disc interface, a sharp blade is utilized to create an annulotomy, and the disc fragments are removed from within the disc space with a pituitary rongeur.
- Step 5
  - A nerve hook is then passed along the inferior, superior, and the foraminal aspects of the nerve root to confirm that no other fragments are present.
  - If there is evidence of foraminal stenosis, a Kerrison rongeur is utilized to remove any foraminal or extraforaminal osteophytes from the outside-in.

POSTOPERATIVE CARE

Complications

- Recurrent disc herniation (Most common)
- Lumbar spine instability
  - This can be prevented by meticulous assessment of the bony anatomy to prevent violation of the pars interarticularis and an excessive facetectomy during bony resection.
- Neuropraxia
  - This can result from aggressive nerve root retraction. Care must be taken to always retract the nerve with gentle pressure and to minimize retraction time.
- Incidental durotomy
  - In general, with a tight surgical wound closure, the paraspinal muscles reduce the dead space, which tamponade the cerebrospinal fluid leak. Patients should remain on flat bed rest for 24 hours.
  - Alternatively, a combination of fibrin glue and patches can be utilized along with the bed rest.

EXPECTED AND ADVERSE OUTCOMES

- A limited discectomy (microdiscectomy) is associated with a lower incidence of long-term low back and leg pain but a higher incidence of recurrent disc herniation when compared with a more aggressive discectomy (subtotal discectomy).[1]
- It is unclear whether a minimally invasive discectomy provides an advantage over an open microsurgical discectomy with respect to the need for admission, length of stay, estimated blood loss, and postoperative narcotic utilization.[2,3]
- A minimally invasive and open discectomy have similar clinical outcomes and complication rates, but the minimally invasive approach may be associated with lower costs.[4]
- A far lateral discectomy is generally associated with good to excellent results. However, recurrent or persistent leg pain has been reported in 21.7% of the cases.[5]

REFERENCES

1. McGirt MJ, Ambrossi GL, Datoo G, et al. Recurrent disc herniation and long-term back pain after primary lumbar discectomy: review of outcomes reported for limited versus aggressive disc removal. Neurosurgery. 2009;64:338-44; discussion 344-35.
2. German JW, Adamo MA, Hoppenot RG, Blossom JH, Nagle HA. Perioperative results following lumbar discectomy: comparison of minimally invasive discectomy and standard microdiscectomy. Neurosurg Focus 2008;25:E20.
3. Harrington JF, French P. Open versus minimally invasive lumbar microdiscectomy: comparison of operative times, length of hospital stay, narcotic use and complications. Minim Invasive Neurosurg: MIN 2008;51:30-5.
4. Lee P, Liu JC, Fessler RG. Perioperative results following open and minimally invasive single-level lumbar discectomy. J Clin Neurosci: official journal of the Neurosurgical Society of Australasia. 2011;18:1667-70.
5. Chang SB, Lee SH, Ahn Y, Kim JM. Risk factor for unsatisfactory outcome after lumbar foraminal and far lateral microdecompression. Spine. 2006;31:1163-7.

REFERENCE SUMMARY

1. McGirt MJ, Ambrossi GL, Datoo G, et al. Recurrent disc herniation and long-term back pain after primary lumbar discectomy: review of outcomes reported for limited versus aggressive disc removal. Neurosurgery 2009;64:338-44; discussion 344-35.

   Summary: A systematic review of the literature comparing the outcomes between an aggressive discectomy (AD) and a limited discectomy (LD). The authors reported that after an AD there is a greater incidence of long-term recurrent back and leg pain. After an LD there is a greater incidence of recurrent disc herniation.

2. German JW, Adamo MA, Hoppenot RG, Blossom JH, Nagle HA. Perioperative results following lumbar discectomy: comparison of minimally invasive discectomy and standard microdiscectomy. Neurosurgical Focus 2008;25:E20.

   Summary: A retrospective study demonstrating that a minimally invasive discectomy is associated with a small but significantly reduced length of stay, estimated blood loss , postoperative narcotic utilization, and hospital admission rate when compared with an open microdiscectomy.

3. Harrington JF, French P. Open versus minimally invasive lumbar micro-discectomy: comparison of operative times, length of hospital stay, narcotic use and complications. Minimally invasive neurosurgery: MIN 2008;51:30-35.

   Summary: A short-term outcome analysis demonstrating that there were no differences in the surgical times, blood loss, complications, and outcomes between a minimally invasive and open microdiscectomy. However, the minimally invsasive cohort demonstrated a shorter length of stay and required less pain medication.

4. Lee P, Liu JC, Fessler RG. Perioperative results following open and minimally invasive single-level lumbar discectomy. Journal of clinical neuroscience: official journal of the Neurosurgical Society of Australasia 2011;18:1667-70.

   Summary: A retrospective analysis demonstarting that a minimally invasive tubular discectomy resulted in a small but statistically significant advantage in length of stay compared with an open microdiscectomy. The authors concluded that this difference may translate into substantial economic savings considering that large number of discectomies that are performed nationally.

5. Chang SB, Lee SH, Ahn Y, Kim JM. Risk factor for unsatisfactory outcome after lumbar foraminal and far lateral microdecompression. Spine 2006;31: 1163-67.

   Summary: The risk factors for unsatisfactory outcomes after a far lateral discectomy were analyzed. After an average follow-up period of 38.4 months, 21.7% (40/184) of the patients reported recurrent or persistent leg pain. The authors concluded that patients with a double herniation were almost three times more likely to have persistent or recurrent leg pain.

Chapter

9

Minimally Invasive Transforaminal Lumbar Interbody Fusion

Alejandro Marquez-Lara, Junyoung Ahn, Kern Singh

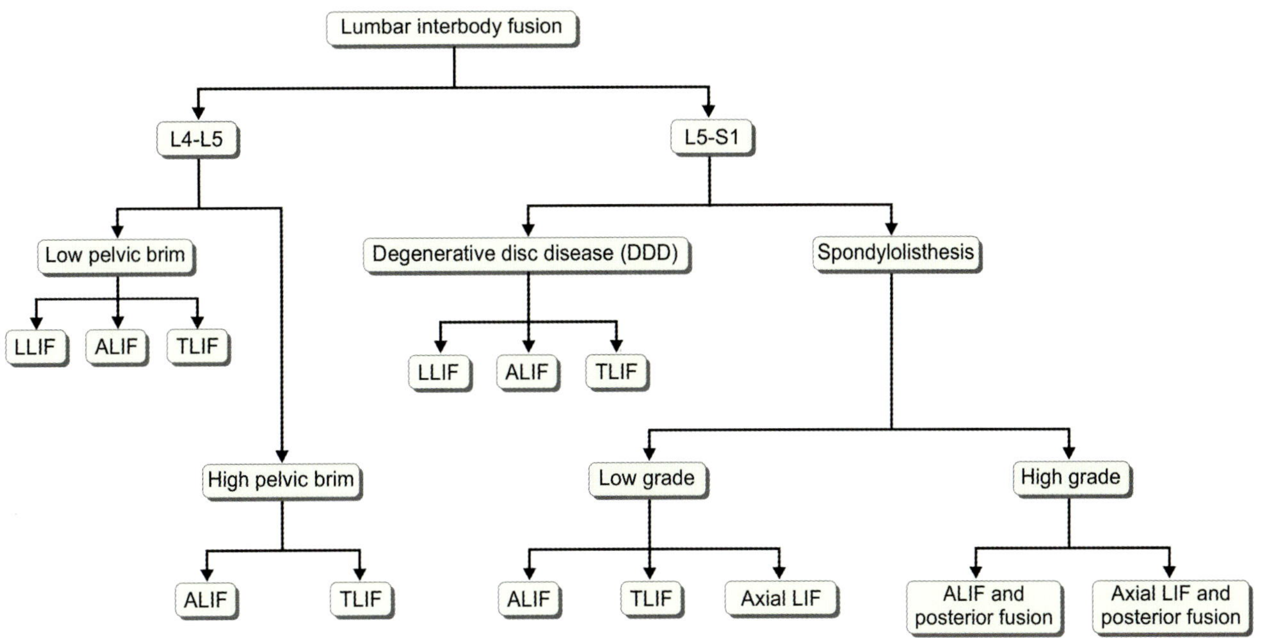

CASE VIGNETTE

A 64-year-old woman with a history of persistent low back pain presents to the clinic with intermittent claudication and worsening right leg pain. The patient denies any bowel or bladder symptoms. On physical examination, there is bilateral lower extremity weakness specifically in the right quadriceps and tibialis anterior muscles. The patient also demonstrates diminished sensation to light touch in the posterior-lateral thighs bilaterally.

DIAGNOSTIC IMAGING

- Plain film radiograph-Anteroposterior (AP) and lateral (Figs. 9.1A and B)
  - Dynamic and static films will help assess the presence and degree of instability.
  - Plain films provide an initial assessment for facet hypertrophy and disc space collapse.

Imaging Pearls

- For recurrent symptoms, the stenosis typically remains in the lateral recess and foramen.

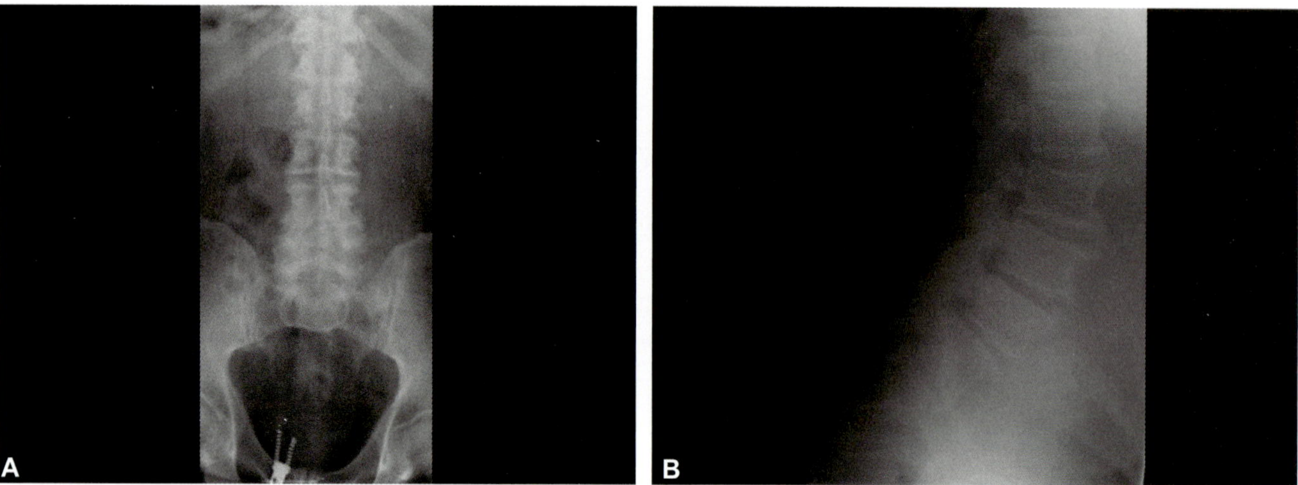

Figs. 9.1A and B: Preoperative (A) anteroposterior and (B) lateral radiographs demonstrating degenerative changes and, low-grade spondylolisthesis at L4–L5.

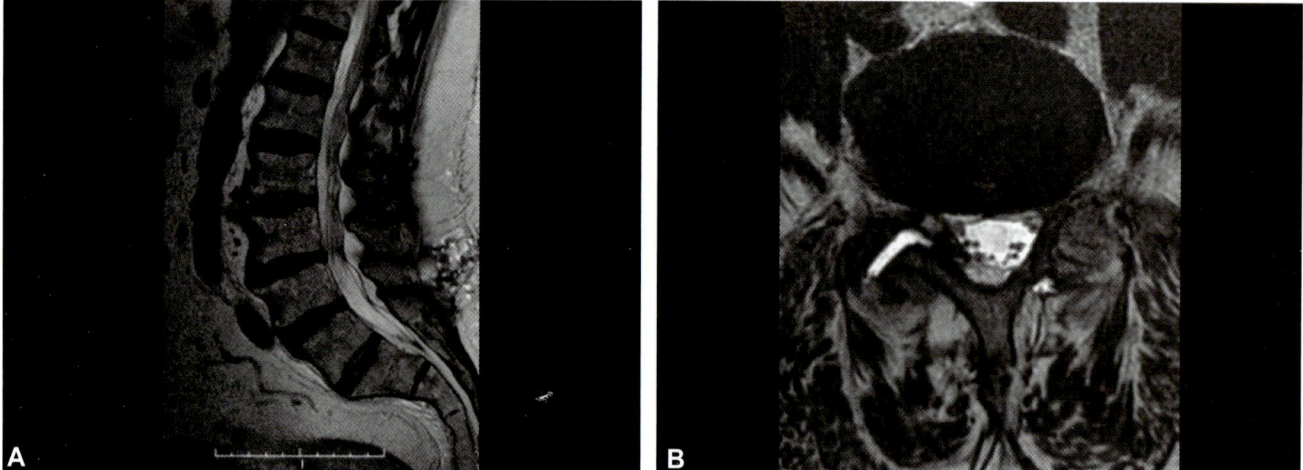

Figs. 9.2A and B: Preoperative (A) sagittal and (B) axial magnetic resonance imaging demonstrating degenerative changes with a right L4-5 facet cyst and facet fluid suggestive of a spondylolisthesis.

- Magnetic resonance imaging (Figs. 9.2A and B)
  - Confirms the presence of a hypertrophic facet fluid
  - Enables the surgeon to determine the diameter and length of the lumbar pedicles
  - Helps plan the anatomical placement of the tubular retractor

SURGICAL INDICATIONS

- Spondylolisthesis-Grade I-II
  - Degenerative
  - Isthmic
- Spinal stenosis
- Recurrent symptomatic disc herniation
- Postlaminectomy instability
- Trauma
- Pseudarthrosis

Indication Controversies

- High-grade spondylolisthesis
  - Dysplasia
- Discogenic surgery

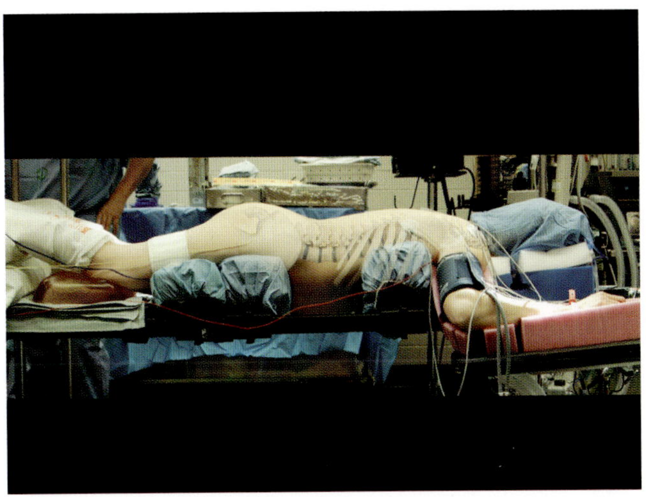

Fig. 9.3: The patient is placed prone on a Jackson table. Note the chest pad is placed just below the axilla to avoid pressure on the brachial plexus. The hip and thigh pads are placed just below the level of the anterior superior iliac spine and gel pads are placed under the patellae. The abdomen is allowed to hang freely to prevent venous congestion.

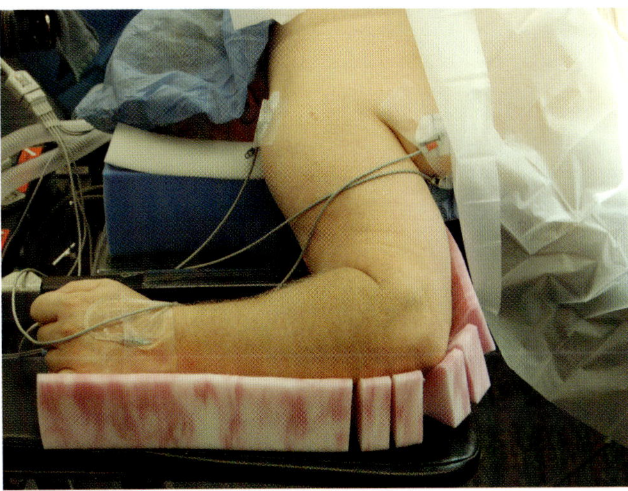

Fig. 9.4: The arms are abducted and the elbows are flexed 90°. A pad is placed under the elbow to prevent compression of the ulnar nerve.

INSTRUMENTATION

- Jackson table
- Surgical loupes or microscope
- Intraoperative fluoroscopy
- Dilators
- Tubular retractor (expandable vs nonexpandable)
- Jamshidi needle
- Hemostatic agents
- Guidewire (Kirschner)
- Interbody spacer/cage
- Pedicle screws
- Rods
- Bone graft
  - Allograft
  - Autograft

POSITIONING AND INTRAOPERATIVE SETUP

- Endotracheal intubation is performed in a supine position.
- Neuromonitoring with electromyography (EMG) testing should be utilized.
- The patient is placed into a prone position on a Jackson table.
  - The abdomen is allowed to hang freely to reduce the intra-abdominal pressure and prevent secondary venous congestion (Fig. 9.3).
- The arms are abducted, elbows are flexed to 90°, and appropriate padding is placed over the bony prominences (Fig. 9.4).
- A chest roll is positioned to maximize lumbar lordosis.
- The surgeon should be positioned on the side of the pathology, while the fluoroscope and monitor are placed on the opposite side of the surgeon.

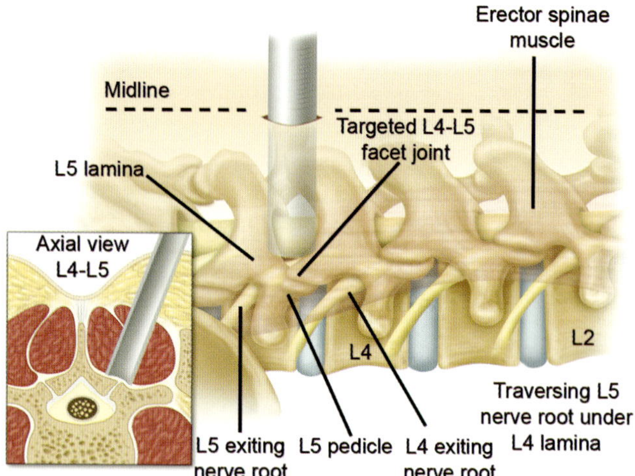

Fig. 9.5: Intraoperative photograph demonstrating the incision site marked just lateral to the midline over the affected level.

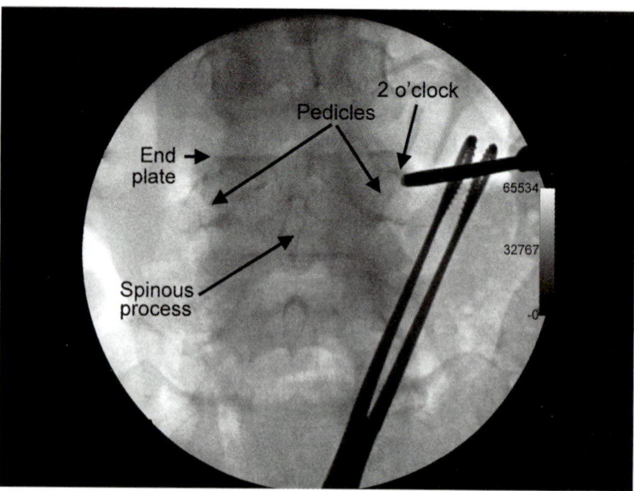

Fig. 9.6: Anteroposterior radiograph demonstrating the correct starting point for the Jamshidi needle at the 2 o'clock position of the right pedicle.

SURGICAL ANATOMY AND EXPOSURE

- Relevant anatomy
  - Lumbar pedicles have a medial angulation from posterior to anterior in the transverse plane that increases from 10°–15° at L1 to 30° at L5.
- Surgical exposure
  - The appropriate level is identified under fluoroscopic guidance.
    - On the AP view, the right and left pedicles should be equidistant from the midline spinous process.
  - On the side of the pathology, a 20-30-mm longitudinal skin incision is made just lateral to the pedicle (Fig. 9.5).
    - This will allow medialization of the Jamshidi needle into the pedicle.
    - Incisions should be made more lateral in obese patients.
    - Care should be taken to avoid a far lateral skin incision as this will make the lumbar decompression more challenging.
  - On the contralateral side (percutaneous pedicle placement only), either stab incisions or a single incision can be made.

PROCEDURE-SPECIFIC STEPS

- Step 1
  - The Jamshidi needle is advanced through the fascia and paraspinal musculature until reaching the starting point of the pedicle (Fig. 9.6).
    - The starting point is at the junction of the transverse process and the facet complex.
      - The correct starting point is at the 2 o'clock position on the right pedicle and 10 o'clock position on the left pedicle in the AP fluoroscopic image.

Step 1 Pearls

- If cannulation of the pedicle is difficult (hypertrophic facet) or if the integrity of the pedicle is questioned (the guidewire does not pass easily or there is a positive EMG stimulation response), a provisional tubular retractor can be placed over the guidewire at the superior facet. Direct visualization can confirm the starting point while still utilizing the percutaneous technique.

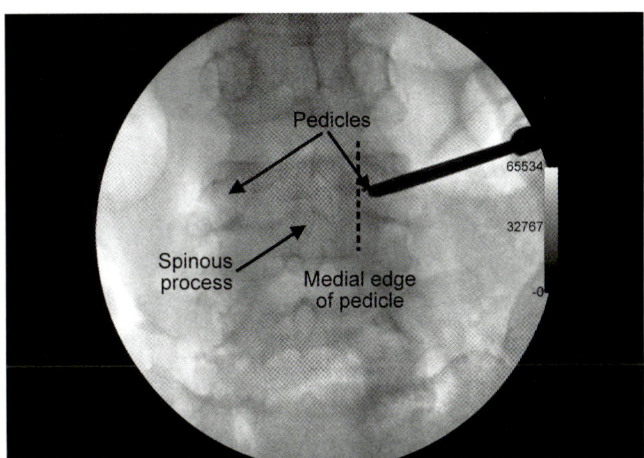

Fig. 9.7: The Jamshidi needle is advanced slowly ensuring that the medial edge of the pedicle is not violated.

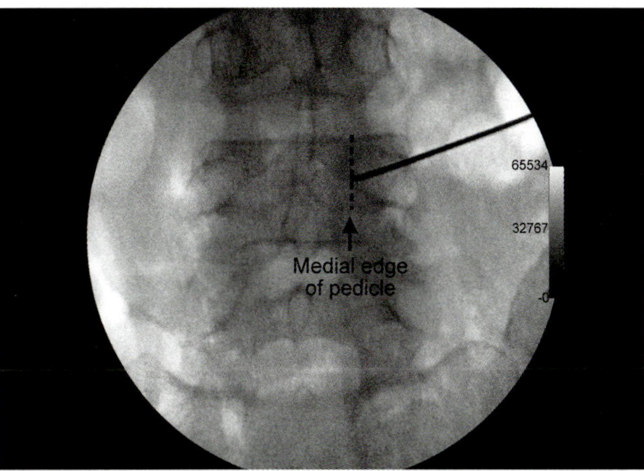

Fig. 9.8: Anteroposterior fluoroscopy demonstrating a guidewire that has been advanced through the Jamshidi needle while maintaining the integrity of the medial wall of the pedicle.

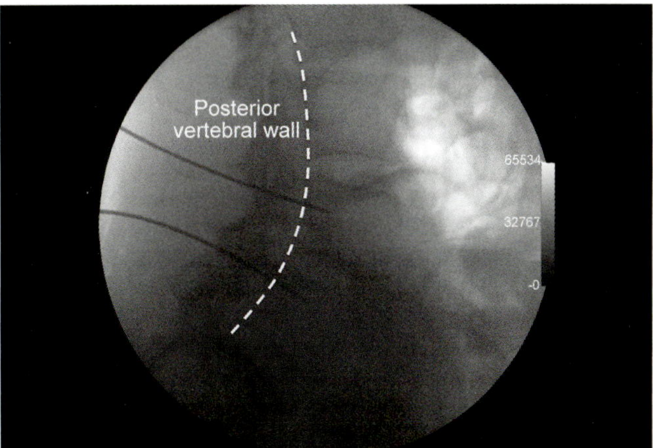

Fig. 9.9: A lateral fluoroscopy demonstrating guidewires that have been advanced beyond the posterior wall of the vertebral body.

- Step 2
  - The Jamshidi needle is advanced in 5-mm increments into the pedicle under AP fluoroscopic guidance.
    - Caution must be taken to avoid crossing the medial edge of the pedicle (Fig. 9.7).
  - After advancing the Jamshidi needle 15–20 mm into the pedicle, a guidewire is placed into the shaft until the tip of the guidewire reaches the medial wall of the pedicle in the AP fluoroscopic view (Fig. 9.8).
  - A lateral view is then obtained to confirm that the tip of the guidewire has crossed the posterior wall of the vertebral body (Fig. 9.9).
    - If the guidewire does not cross the posterior wall of the vertebral body on the lateral view or if it crosses the medial wall of the pedicle in the AP view, the Jamshidi needle should be redirected to a more lateral trajectory.

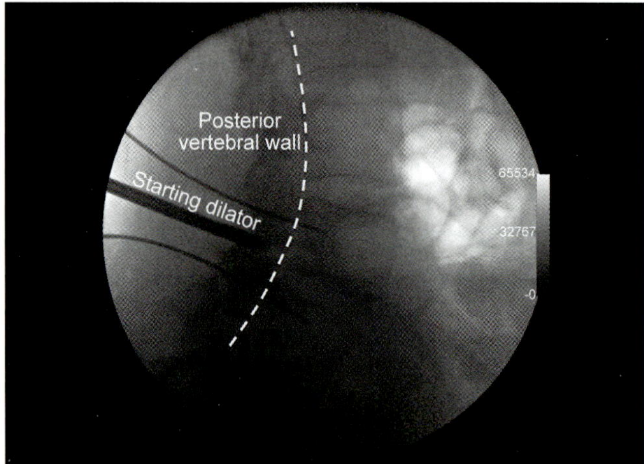

Fig. 9.10: A starting dilator is inserted between the guidewires creating a working channel to access the intervertebral disc space while minimizing soft tissue dissection.

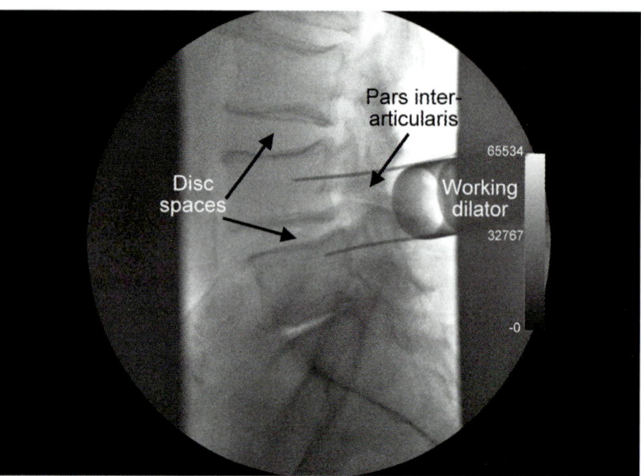

Fig. 9.11: Lateral fluoroscopy demonstrating the final position of the self-retaining retractor at the target level.

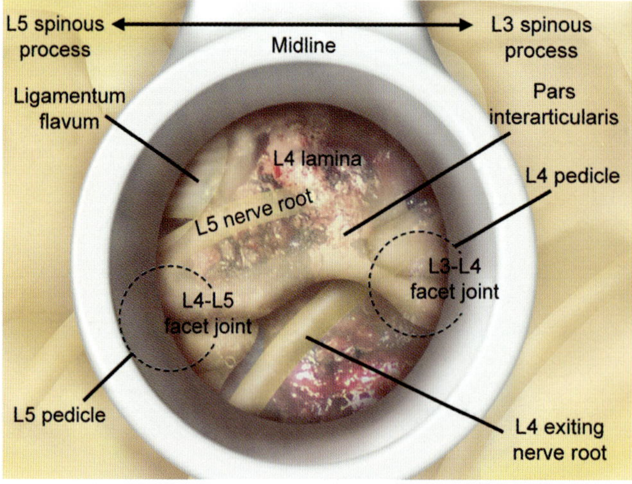

Fig. 9.12: Intraoperative view of the surgical working channel.

- Step 3
  - After cannulating the pedicles above and below the level of fusion, an initial dilator is passed between the guidewires (Fig. 9.10).
  - Sequential dilation is performed, and a tubular retractor is docked onto the pars interarticularis at the disc space level (Fig. 9.11).
  - The remaining muscle and soft tissue is removed with electrocautery and rongeurs for adequate visualization (Fig. 9.12).
- Step 4
  - A high-speed burr is utilized to remove the lamina and the inferior facet of the cephalad vertebrae (Fig. 9.13A). The laminectomy is extended superiorly to the insertion of the ligamentum flavum and laterally through the pars interarticularis.
  - The inferior articular process of the cephalad vertebrae is then removed to complete the facetectomy (Fig. 9.13B).
    - If bilateral decompression is necessary, the spinous process can be undercut to enable the contralateral laminectomy and facetectomy.

Step 3 Pearls

- The retractor should be centered over the facet joint with a parallel and medial trajectory to the disc space.

Step 4 Pearls

- Inadequate resection of the facet joint will reduce the visualization of the disc space. This may result in the placement of an undersized cage, thus increasing the likelihood of cage migration and pseudarthrosis.

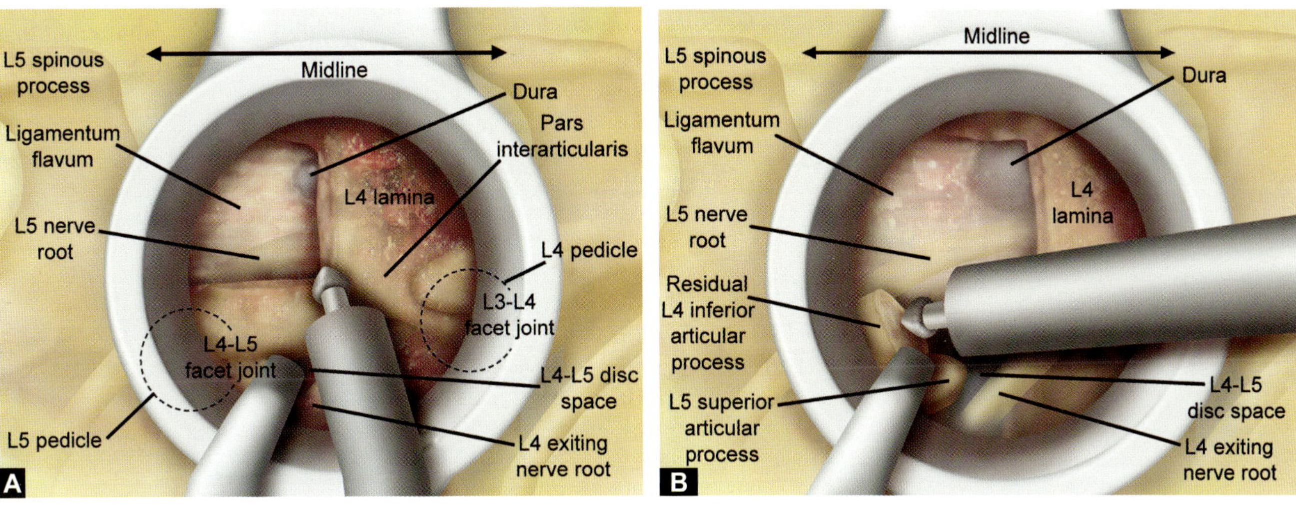

Figs. 9.13A and B: A high-speed burr is utilized to remove the (A) lamina, (B) part of the facet, and inferior articular process of the cephalad vertebrae.

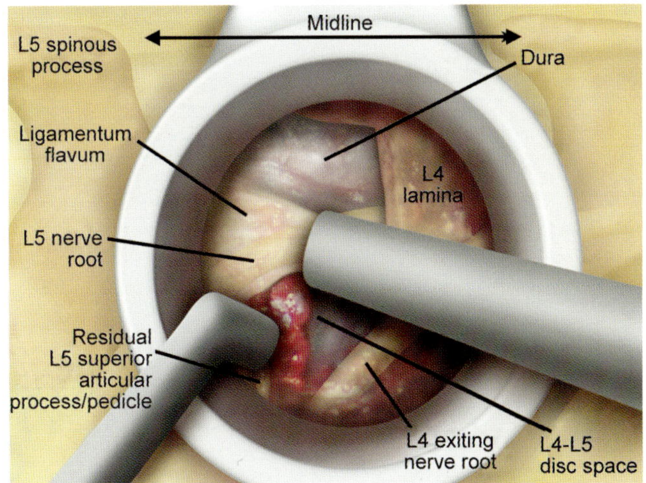

Fig. 9.14: A Kerrison rongeur is used to remove the ligamentum flavum in order to expose the traversing and exiting nerve roots.

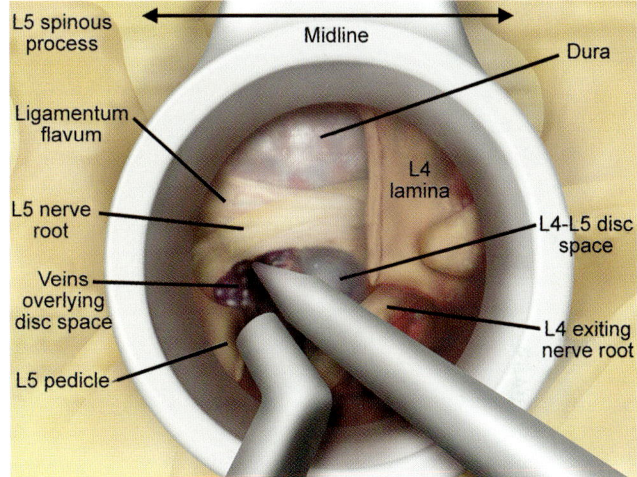

Fig. 9.15: Bipolar cautery is utilized to coagulate the veins that overly the disc space.

  - The ligamentum flavum, which is left intact to protect the dura during the facetectomy, is then removed with a Kerrison rongeur. This will expose the traversing and exiting nerve roots (Fig. 9.14).
- Step 5
  - The intervertebral disc space is identified and bipolar electrocautery is utilized to coagulate the veins that overlie the disc (Fig. 9.15).
  - After adequately protecting the neural structures, an annulotomy is then performed with a no.15 blade.
  - A Kerrison rongeur can be utilized within the annulotomy to release the posterior longitudinal ligament (PLL) as far to the contralateral side as possible.
    - This facilitates visualization and increases the mobility of the disc space for distraction.

Step 5 Pearls

- It is important to resect the entire superior articular process at the L5-S1 level to lateralize the tubular dilator starting point while medializing its trajectory.

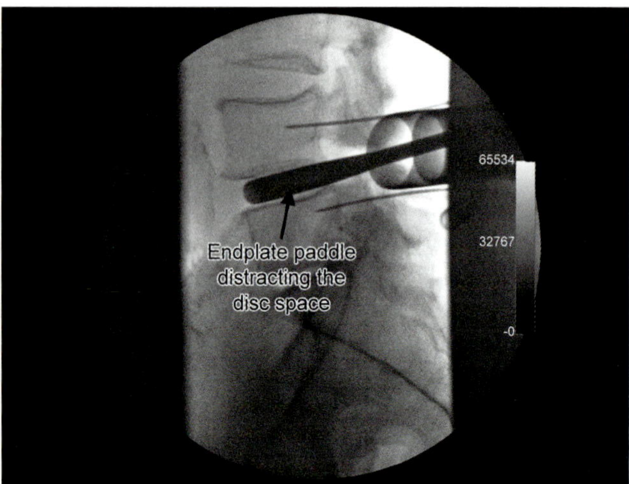

Fig. 9.16: Intraoperative lateral fluoroscopy demonstrating the preparation of the intervertebral disc space for implant placement.

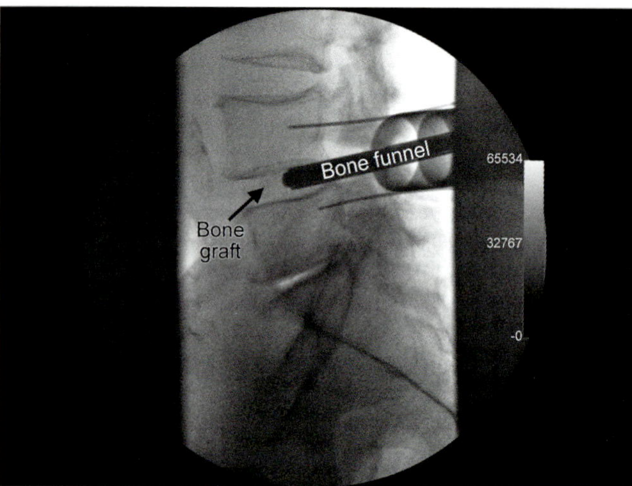

Fig. 9.17: Intraoperative lateral fluoroscopy demonstrating a bone funnel in the disc space, which allows insertion of graft material.

- Step 6
  - A subtotal discectomy is then performed with a combination of disc shavers, pituitary rongeurs, and curved curettes.
    - If necessary, contralateral pedicle screws can be placed to distract the disc space for further instrumentation.
  - The disc space is then prepared with paddle distractors, curettes, and endplate shavers under lateral fluoroscopic guidance (Fig. 9.16).
- Step 7
  - After preparing the endplates, a trial interbody cage is placed through a bone funnel and sized to restore the appropriate lumbar lordosis.
  - The trial cage is then removed and the disc space is copiously irrigated and cleared of any debris.
- Step 8
  - Morcellized autologous bone graft saved from the laminectomy and facetectomy is packed in the anterior disc space and/or in the interbody cage (Fig. 9.17).
  - The intervertebral cage is advanced under fluoroscopic guidance with care to protect the traversing nerve root (Figs. 9.18A and B).
- Step 9
  - With the cage in place, the pedicle screws can then be placed.
  - A pedicle tap is advanced over the guidewire until it crosses the posterior vertebral body wall (Fig. 9.19).
    - The tap can be stimulated with EMG-evoked potentials.
- Step 10
  - The tap is removed over the guidewire and a cannulated pedicle screw of the appropriate length, and diameter is then inserted under fluoroscopic guidance (Fig. 9.20).
  - After screw placement, an AP and lateral fluoroscopic view should be obtained to assess the screw positioning.

Step 6 Pearls

- If the disc space is extremely collapsed, the PLL should be released as far across the midline as possible and the contralateral facet should be released as well.
- If the nerve root is overlying the disc space, the superior portion of the inferior pedicle can be removed to gain access to the disc caudal to the root.

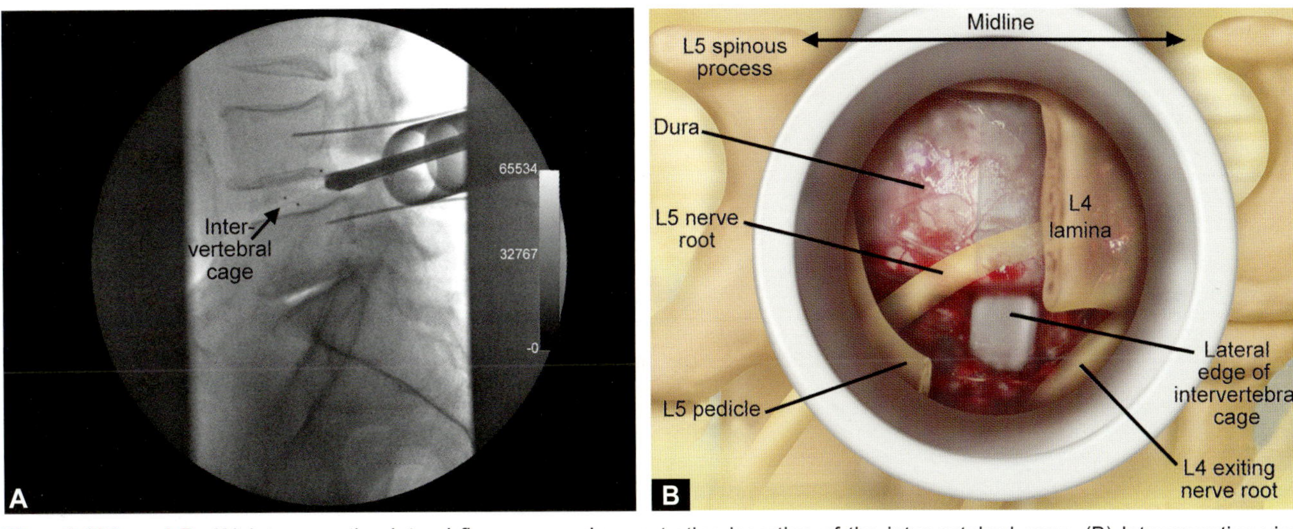

Figs. 9.18A and B: (A) Intraoperative lateral fluoroscopy demonstrating insertion of the intervertebral cage. (B) Intraoperative view of the intervertebral cage through the surgical working channel.

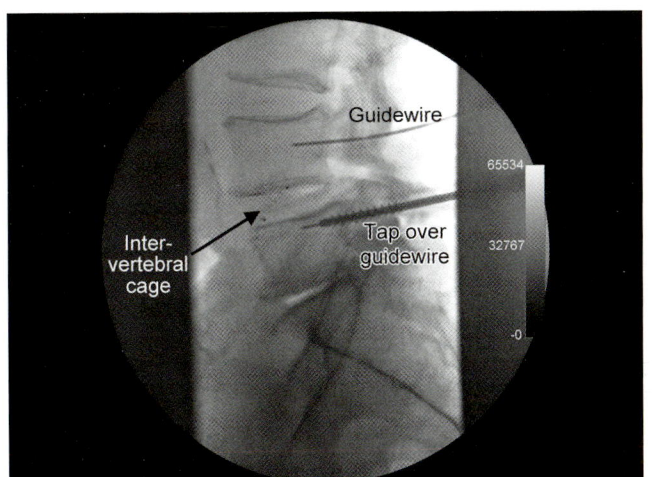

Fig. 9.19: Lateral fluoroscopy utilized to visualize the pedicle tap being placed over the guidewire.

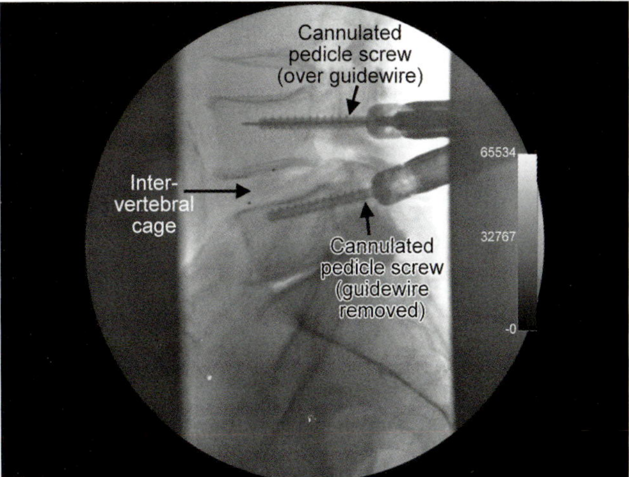

Fig. 9.20: Insertion of cannulated pedicle screws over the guidewire above and below the target disc space.

- Step 11
  - An appropriately sized rod is then inserted submuscularly through the screw slots and compression is applied across the intervertebral graft (Figs. 9.21A and B).

POSTOPERATIVE CARE

Complications

- Incidental durotomies
  - Most can be treated conservatively with a collagen sponge and fibrin glue followed by 24 hours of bed rest.

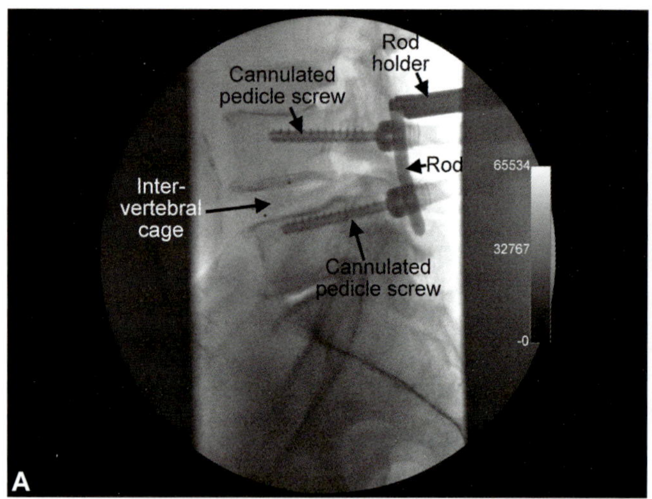

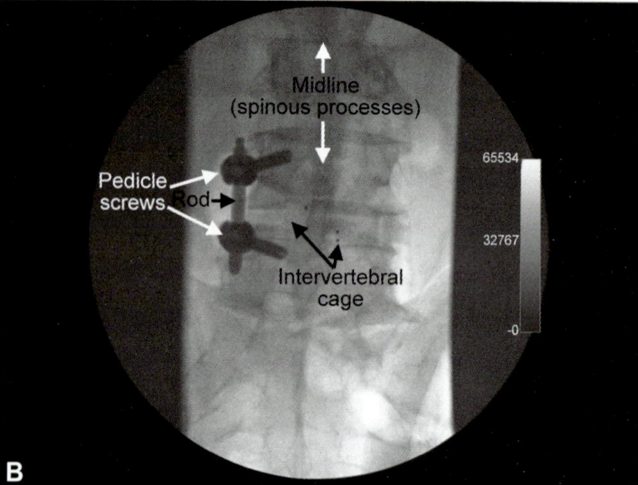

Figs. 9.21A and B: (B) Lateral fluoroscopy confirming the rod has been placed through the screw heads. (B) Anteroposterior fluoroscopy of the final construct.

- Screw malposition
  - Medial pedicle wall breach
  - Surgical site infection
  - Extradural hematoma
  - Persistent radiculopathy

EXPECTED AND ADVERSE OUTCOMES

- Compared with an open approach, a minimally invasive transforaminal lumbar interbody fusion (TLIF) carries a shorter operative and anesthesia time as well as a reduced blood loss, hospital stay, and total hospital costs.[1]
- A minimally invasive TLIF is associated with reduced narcotic pain medication requirements and a quicker return to work.[2,3]
- The risk of surgical site infection is significantly reduced with a minimally invasive TLIF when compared with an open approach.[4]
- At 6-month follow-up, minimally invasive TLIF-treated patients can expect a 94.8% arthrodesis rate of up which is similar to that of an open TLIF (90.1%).[5]

REFERENCES

1. Pelton MA, Phillips FM, Singh K. A comparison of perioperative costs and outcomes in patients with and without workers' compensation claims treated with minimally invasive or open transforaminal lumbar interbody fusion. Spine (Phila Pa 1976). 2012;37:1914-9.
2. Adogwa O, Parker SL, Bydon A, Cheng J, McGirt MJ. Comparative effectiveness of minimally invasive versus open transforaminal lumbar interbody fusion–2-year assessment of narcotic use, return to work, disability, and quality of life. J Spinal Disord Tech. 2011;24:479-84.
3. Parker SL, Lerner J, McGirt MJ. Effect of minimally invasive technique on return to work and narcotic use following transforaminal lumbar inter-body fusion: a review. Prof Case Manag. 2012;17:229-35.

4. Parker SL, Adogwa O, Witham TF, et al. Post-operative infection after minimally invasive versus open transforaminal lumbar interbody fusion (TLIF): literature review and cost analysis. Minim Invasive Neurosurg: MIN. 2011;54:33-7.
5. Wu RH, Fraser JF, Hartl R. Minimal access versus open transforaminal lumbar interbody fusion—meta-analysis of fusion rates. Spine. 2010;35:2273-81.

REFERENCE SUMMARY

1. Pelton MA, Phillips FM, Singh K. A comparison of perioperative costs and outcomes in patients with and without workers' compensation claims treated with minimally invasive or open transforaminal lumbar interbody fusion. Spine (Phila Pa 1976). 2012;37:1914-9.
   Summary: A prospective review comparing the outcomes of patients undergoing either an open or MIS TLIF with regards to workers' compensation (WC) status. Patients who underwent an MIS TLIF regardless of the WC status demonstrated significantly better short-term outcomes and lower hospital cots than the open TLIF cohort.
2. Adogwa O, Parker SL, Bydon A, Cheng J, McGirt MJ. Comparative Effectiveness of Minimally Invasive Versus Open Transforaminal Lumbar Interbody Fusion—2-year Assessment of Narcotic Use, Return to Work, Disability, and Quality of Life. J Spinal Disord Tech. 2011;24:479-84.
   Summary: A retrospective review of 30 patients who underwent either an open or MIS TLIF. At 2 years after surgery, the MIS TLIF cohort demonstrated a reduced postoperative narcotic requirement and a quicker return to work.
3. Parker SL, Lerner J, McGirt MJ. Effect of minimally invasive technique on return to work and narcotic use following transforaminal lumbar inter-body fusion: a review. Professional Case Management. 2012;17:229-35.
   Summary: A systematic literature review that demonstrates that an MIS TLIF is associated with quicker return to work and narcotic cessation when compared with an open TLIF.
4. Parker SL, Adogwa O, Witham TF, Aaronson OS, Cheng J, McGirt MJ. Post-operative infection after minimally invasive versus open transforaminal lumbar interbody fusion (TLIF): literature review and cost analysis. Minimally Invasive Neurosurgery: MIN. 2011;54:33-7.
   Summary: A systematic review comparing the incidence of postoperative surgical site infection (SSI) after an open or MIS TLIF. The authors demonstrated a lower SSI rate associated with an MIS TLIF, which carried an overall reduction in hospital costs.
5. Wu RH, Fraser JF, Hartl R. Minimal access versus open transforaminal lumbar interbody fusion—meta-analysis of fusion rates. Spine. 2010;35:2273-81.
   Summary: A meta-analysis to compare fusion rates between open and MIS TLIFs. The arthrodesis rates at 6 months are relatively high (>90%) for both approaches. In addition, the complication rates are also similar with a trend toward fewer complications withan MIS TLIF.

Chapter

10

Minimally Invasive Lateral Lumbar Interbody Fusion

Sreeharsha V Nandyala, Branko Skovrlj, Sheeraz A Qureshi, Kern Singh

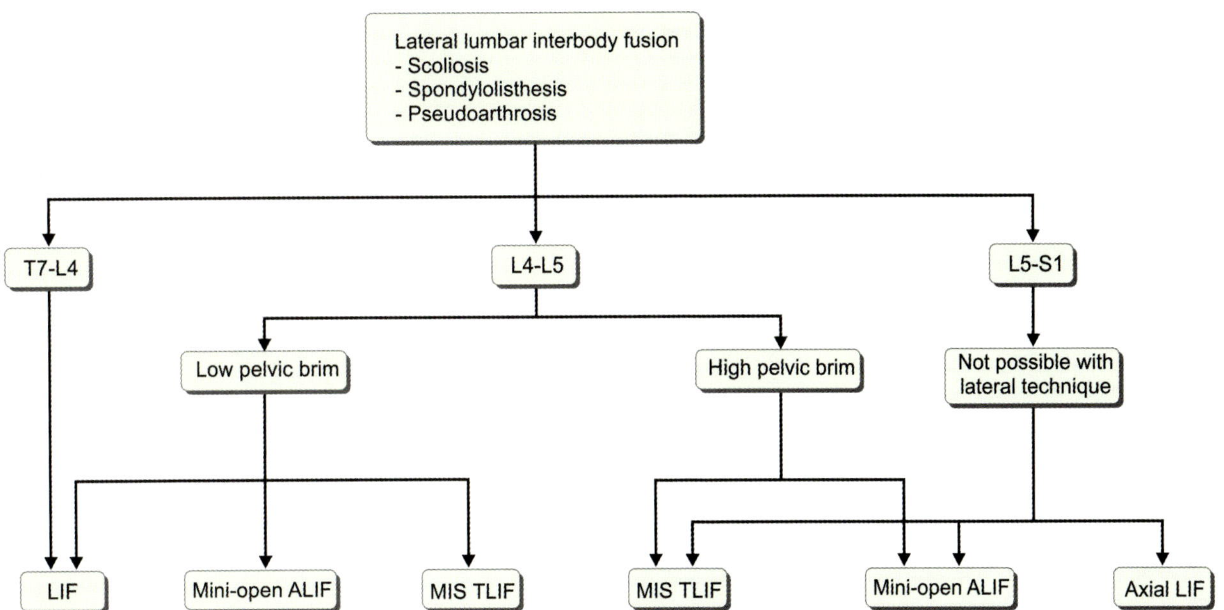

CASE VIGNETTE

A 67-year-old woman presents to the office with low back pain and bilateral lower extremity pain and weakness. Her symptoms worsen after standing or walking and improve with rest. On examination, the patient demonstrates left quadriceps and tibialis anterior weakness, a decrease in the left patellar reflex, and reduced sensation on the anterior aspect of the left knee.

DIAGNOSTIC IMAGING

- Plain film radiograph—Anteroposterior (AP) and lateral (Figs. 10.1A to C)
  - Provides an initial assessment of the disc space, vertebral bodies, degree of degeneration, and stability of the lumbar spine
  - The proximal extent of the iliac crest can determine if access to the L4–L5 interspace is feasible.

Imaging Pearls

- The axial T1 weighted image at the affected level should be evaluated. Within the psoas muscle, the nerve roots can be identified. This preoperative planning can help determine where to dock the initial dilator during the transpsoas approach.

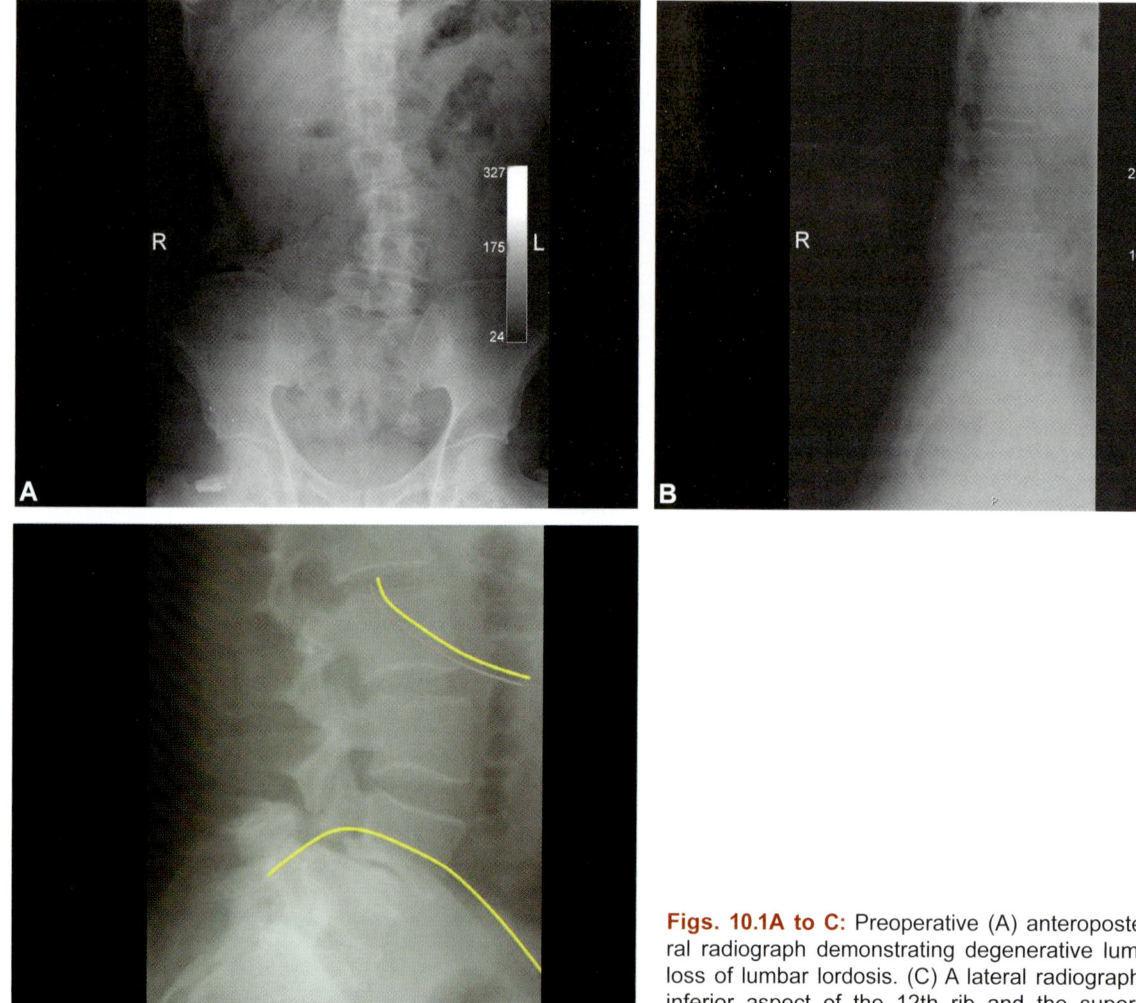

Figs. 10.1A to C: Preoperative (A) anteroposterior and (B) lateral radiograph demonstrating degenerative lumbar scoliosis and loss of lumbar lordosis. (C) A lateral radiograph demarcating the inferior aspect of the 12th rib and the superior aspect of the iliac crest.

- Magnetic resonance imaging (MRI) (Figs. 10.2A to C)
  - MRI is the diagnostic imaging modality of choice to identify and characterize the level and extent of the pathology.
  - Allows the surgeon to establish a safe approach by identifying critical structures including the great vessels, the lumbar plexus, and the psoas muscle
- Computed tomography (CT)
  - In cases where an MRI is contraindicated (ocular implants, cardiac pacemakers, etc.) a CT myelogram can help identify neural compression.

SURGICAL INDICATIONS

- Spinal instability (T7-L4)
- Adjacent segment degeneration
- Pseudarthrosis

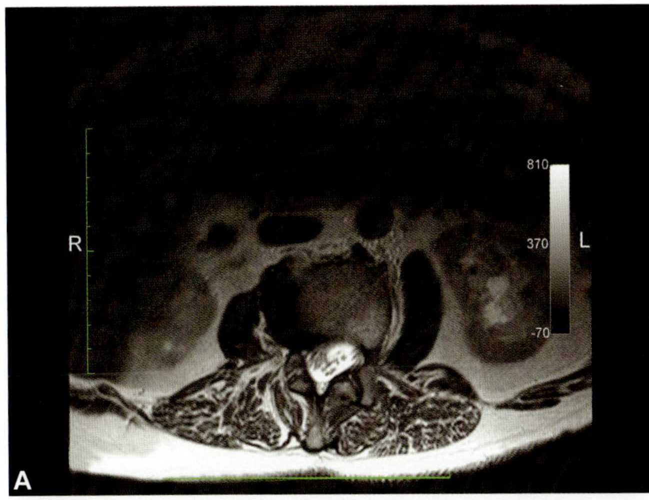

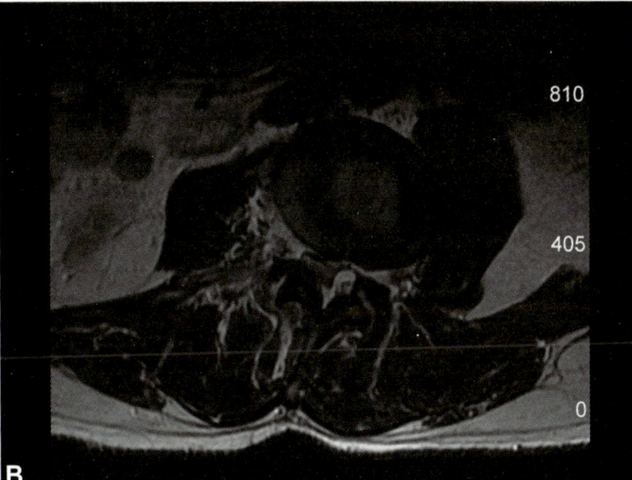

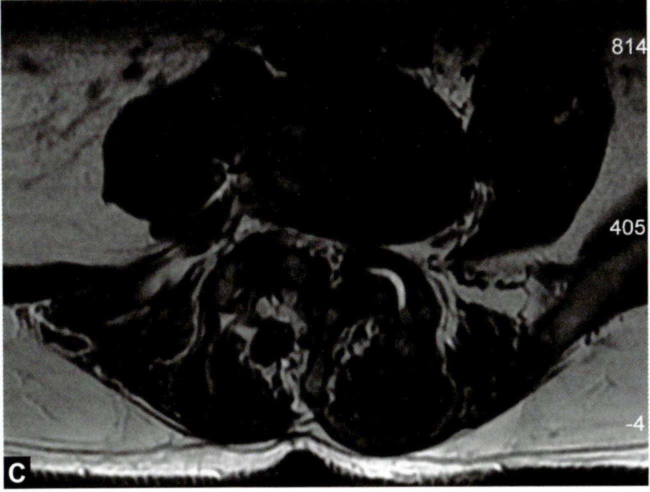

Figs. 10.2A to C: Preoperative magnetic resonance imaging demonstrating degenerative changes and spinal stenosis at (A) L2–L3, (B) L3–L4, and (C) L4–L5.

- Degenerative conditions
  - Spondylosis with stenosis
  - Scoliosis
  - Degenerative disc disease
- Spondylolisthesis (Grade I–II)
- Postlaminectomy kyphosis
- Tumors
- Infections

Contraindications

- Grade III–IV spondylolisthesis
- Severe stenosis
- Vascular abnormality

Controversies

- Previous retroperitoneal surgery
- Severely collapsed disc spaces
- Severe osteoporosis may be a contraindication for a stand-alone lateral intervertebral device.

INSTRUMENTATION

- Radiolucent surgical table
- Intraoperative fluoroscopy
- Expandable retractor and table-mounted retractor arm
- Intervertebral disc spacers or cages
- Bone graft
  - Autograft
  - Allograft

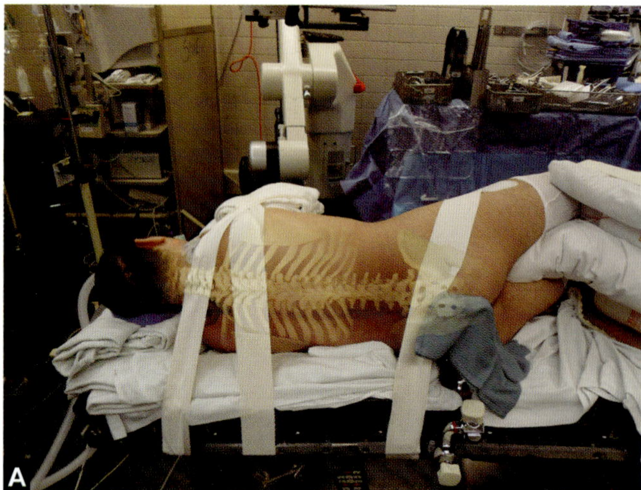

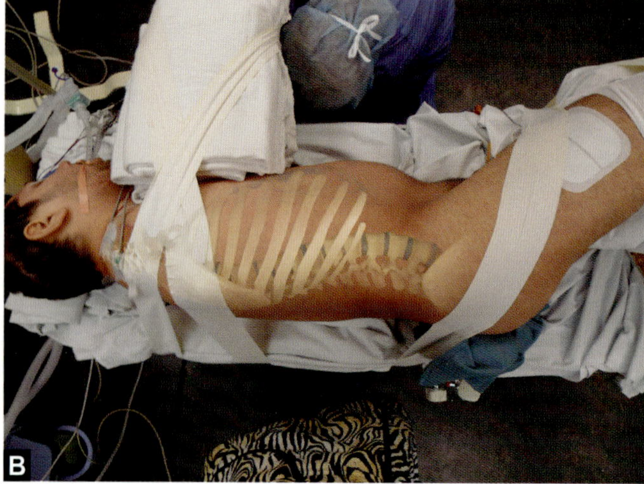

Figs. 10.3A and B: (A) The patient is well secured in a lateral decubitus position with a bump underneath the affected level and the table slightly flexed to increase the distance between the 12th rib and the iliac crest. (B) The patient is positioned with the operative site over the break in the bed to allow maximal flexion at the surgical level.

- Bone graft substitutes
  - Demineralized bone matrices
  - Synthetic products
  - Bone morphogenetic proteins
  - Mesenchymal stem cell containing products
- Shavers
- Curettes
- Rasps
- Cobb elevators

POSITIONING AND INTRAOPERATIVE SETUP

- Neuromonitoring with continuous electromyography (EMG) testing should be utilized when traversing the psoas muscle.
- The patient is placed in a lateral decubitus position. The table should be minimally flexed to increase the distance between the iliac crest and the rib cage (Figs. 10.3A and B).
  - For scoliosis correction, an approach from the concavity may enable access to a greater number of levels from a smaller incision.
  - Care should be taken to identify the proximity of the great vessels, which should be a major determinant of the approach.
- The legs/hips should be flexed to relax the psoas muscle.
- Appropriate padding is placed over the bony prominences.
- An axillary roll is positioned under the dependent axilla, and the pelvis and upper thorax are taped to secure the patient.
- The surgeon should stand posterior to the patient, while the fluoroscopy, monitor, and the mounted retractor arm should be on the opposite side of the surgeon.

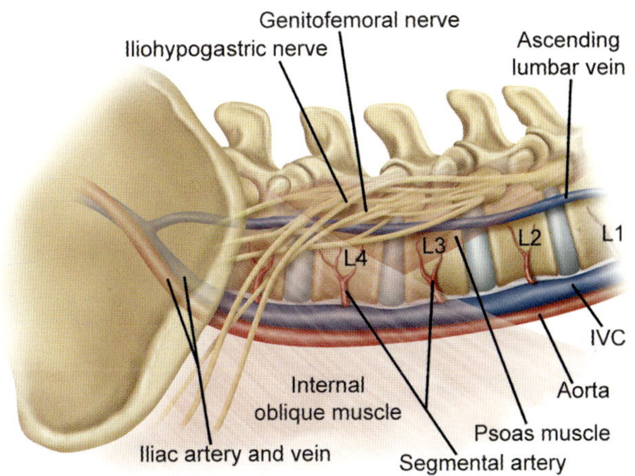

Fig. 10.4: Topographic anatomy of important vascular and neural structures that may be encountered during a lateral lumbar approach.

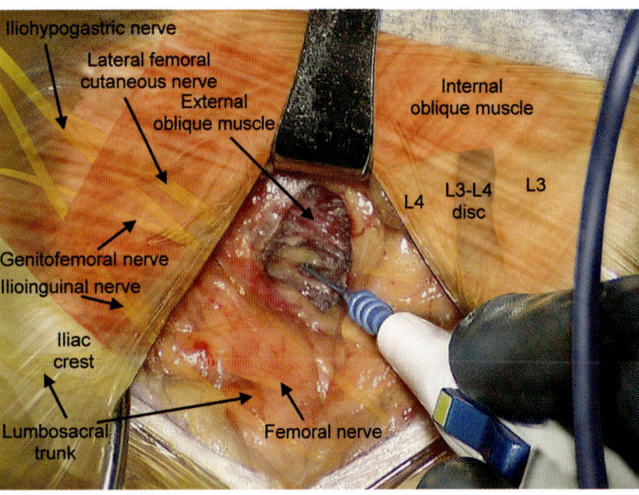

Fig. 10.5: The incision site is marked over the affected disc space (L4–L5) and the skin incision is made exposing the fibers of the external oblique muscle.

SURGICAL ANATOMY AND EXPOSURE

- Relevant anatomy (Fig. 10.4)
  - The nerves of the lumbar plexus traverse dorsally near the posterior endplate of L1–L2. As the nerves descend within the psoas muscle, there is a progressive ventral migration from L2–L3 to L4–L5. Instrumentation through the psoas muscle risks injury to the neural structures.
  - The degree of overlap between the retroperitoneal great vessels and the vertebra increases progressively from proximal to distal, which also contributes to the narrowing of the safe working zone.
- Surgical exposure
  - Under lateral fluoroscopic guidance, the level of interest is localized.
  - A 2-4-cm longitudinal skin incision is made that is centered over the target disc space (Fig. 10.5).
  - The external and internal obliques are split parallel to their muscle fibers, thereby exposing the transversalis fascia (Figs. 10.6A and B).
    - A Kocher clamp is utilized to puncture through the transversalis fascia to enter into the retroperitoneal space (Fig. 10.7).
  - The retroperitoneal fat is retracted anteriorly exposing the psoas muscle.
    - The genitofemoral nerve, coursing on the lateral aspect of the psoas muscles, should be identified and protected.
  - The psoas muscle is then retracted posteriorly or traversed under continuous neuromonitoring (Figs. 10.8A and B).
    - Care must be taken to minimally open the retractor to reduce the likelihood for neurological injury.
    - A neuromonitoring probe should be utilized to determine if any nerve fibers are crossing the surgical field.[1]

Exposure Pearls

- Up to three levels can be accessed through a single incision.

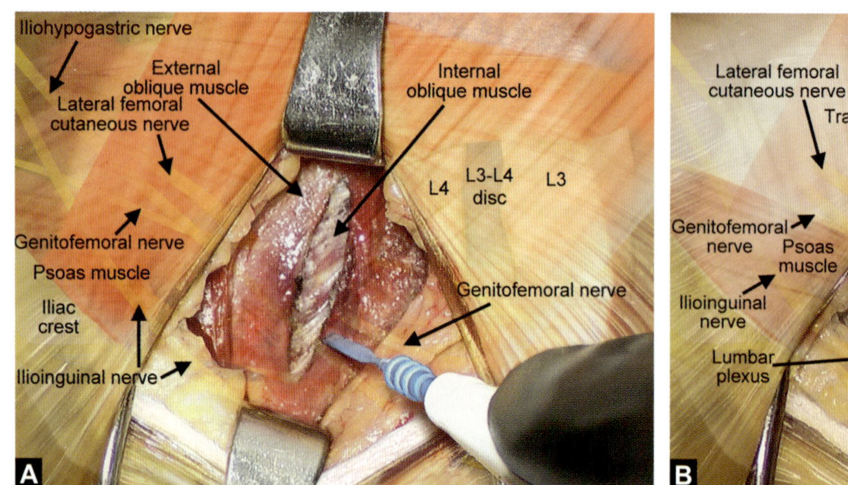

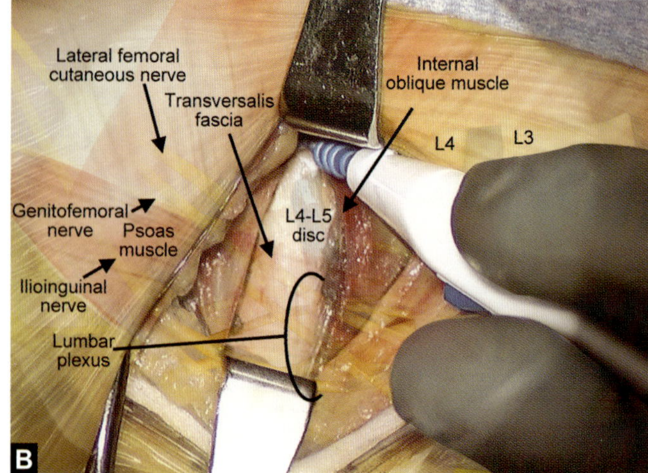

Figs. 10.6A and B: (A) Intraoperative photograph after incision of the external oblique muscle, parallel to its fibers, exposing the internal oblique. (B) After incision of the internal oblique, the transverse fascia is exposed.

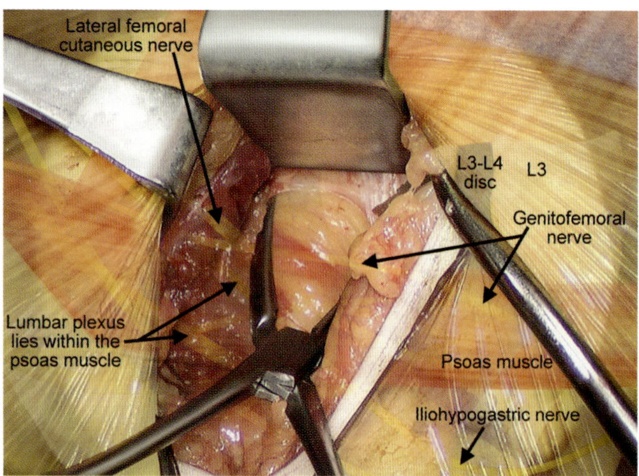

Fig. 10.7: The transversalis fascia is bluntly dissected to expose the retroperitoneal fat.

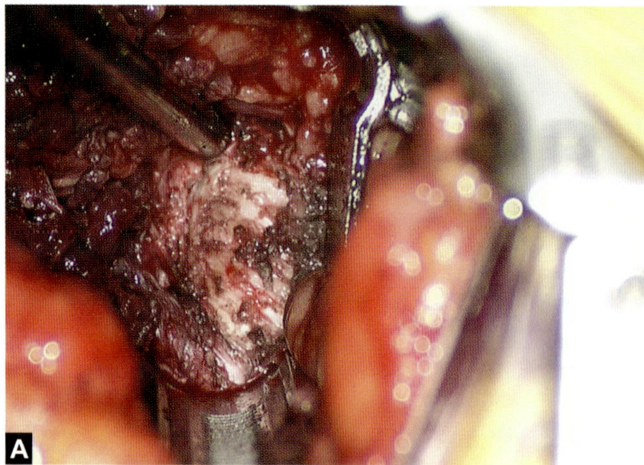

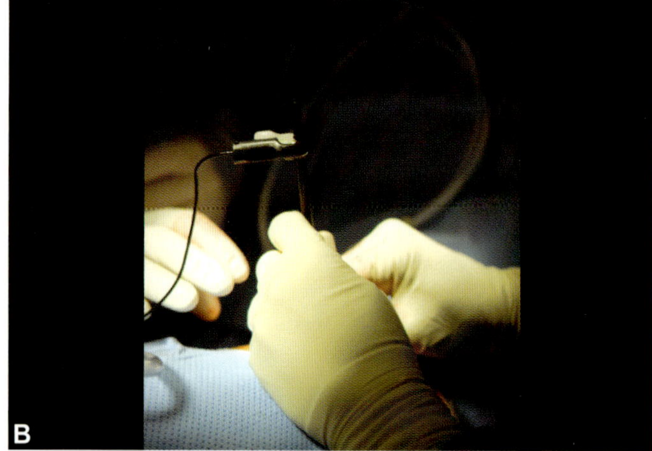

Figs. 10.8A and B: Intraoperative photograph (A) demonstrating anterior retraction of retroperitoneal fat and posterior retraction of the psoas muscles to expose the target level (L4–L5). (B) Neuromonitoring probe docked on the disc space of interest.

PROCEDURE-SPECIFIC STEPS

- Step 1
  - A lateral annulotomy is then performed, and the endplates are prepared utilizing a combination of shavers, curettes, and rasps (Figs. 10.9A to C).
  - Care must be taken to leave the anterior annulus intact.
- Step 2
  - After the discectomy is complete, the contralateral annulus is released with a Cobb elevator to facilitate the correction of deformity in the coronal plane (Fig. 10.10)
    - Care must be taken to minimally advance beyond the contralateral annulus as this increases the risk for nerve injury.
    - Extreme care is taken to not violate the endplate as this dramatically increases the risk of cage subsidence particularly in cases of stand-alone cage utilization.

Procedure Pitfalls

- The iliac crest may limit the surgical exposure to the L4–L5 level.
- The precision of this lateral approach relies heavily upon fluoroscopic guidance, which exposes the surgeon and the patient to high doses of radiation.

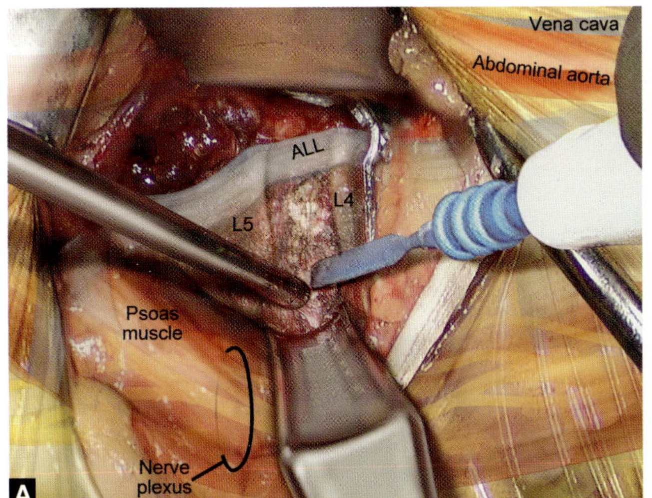

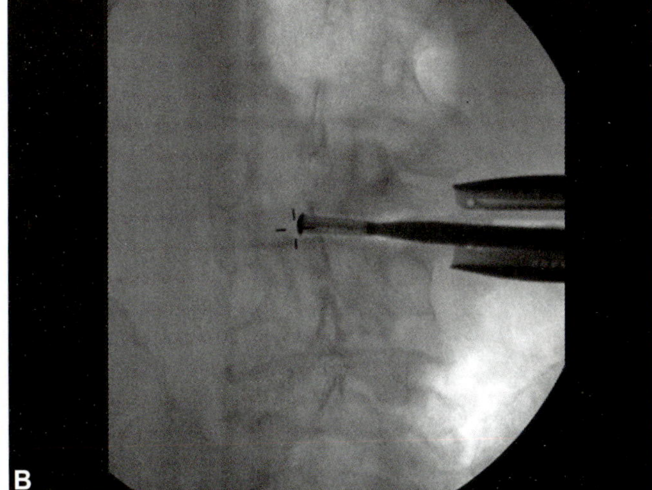

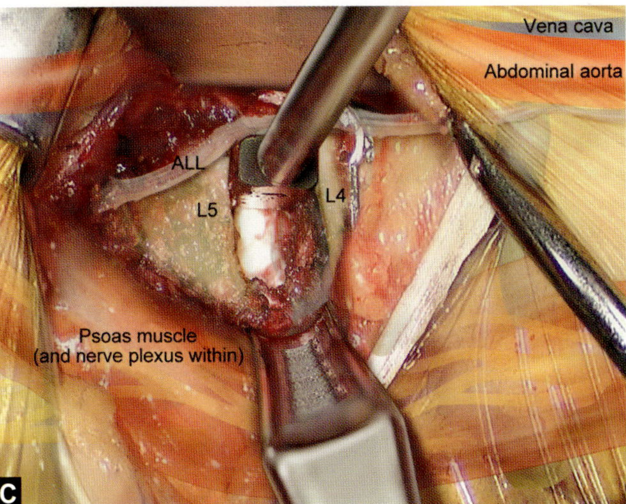

Figs. 10.9A to C: (A) A lateral annulotomy is performed while protecting the neural structures behind the retractor. (B) Discectomy is performed with a series of shavers and curettes under intraoperative fluoroscopy. (C) The endplates are then prepared with care not to violate the endplates.

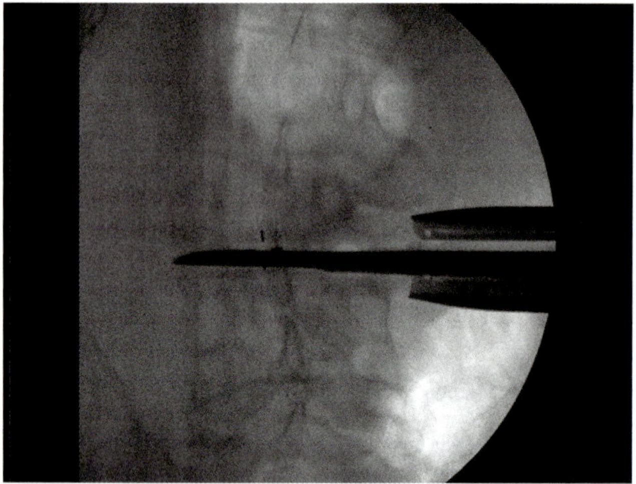

Fig. 10.10: Intraoperative anteroposterior fluoroscopy demonstrating release of the contralateral annulus with a Cobb elevator.

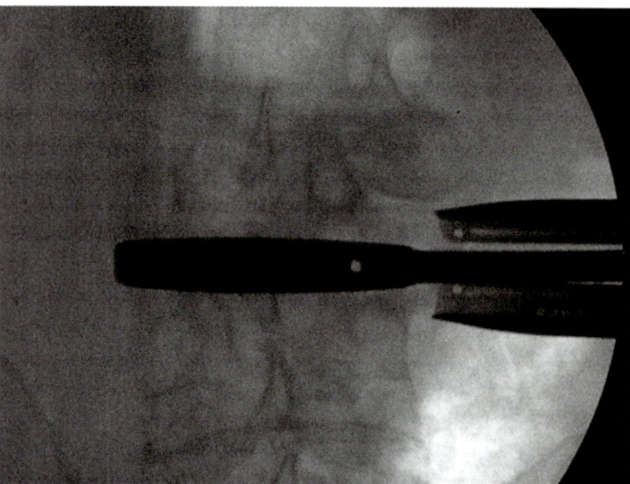

Fig. 10.11: Intraoperative anteroposterior fluoroscopy of a trial implant that helps determine the length and height of the final implant.

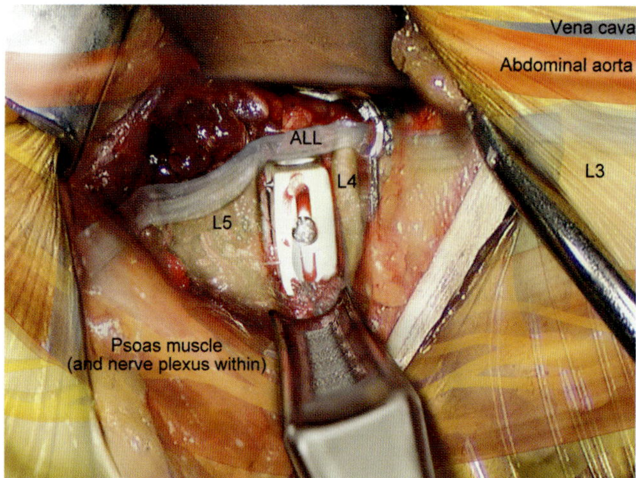

Fig. 10.12: The final implant is gently impacted into place.

- Step 3
  - The implant size is then determined with sizers and trials (Fig. 10.11).
    - The cage should be sized such that it just overhangs both sides of the apophyseal ring, allowing maximum weight bearing of the device.
  - The cage is filled with bone graft or bone graft substitute and then impacted across the disc space (Fig. 10.12).
  - Postoperative radiographs (AP and lateral) confirm the final position of the intervertebral cage (Figs. 10.13A and B).

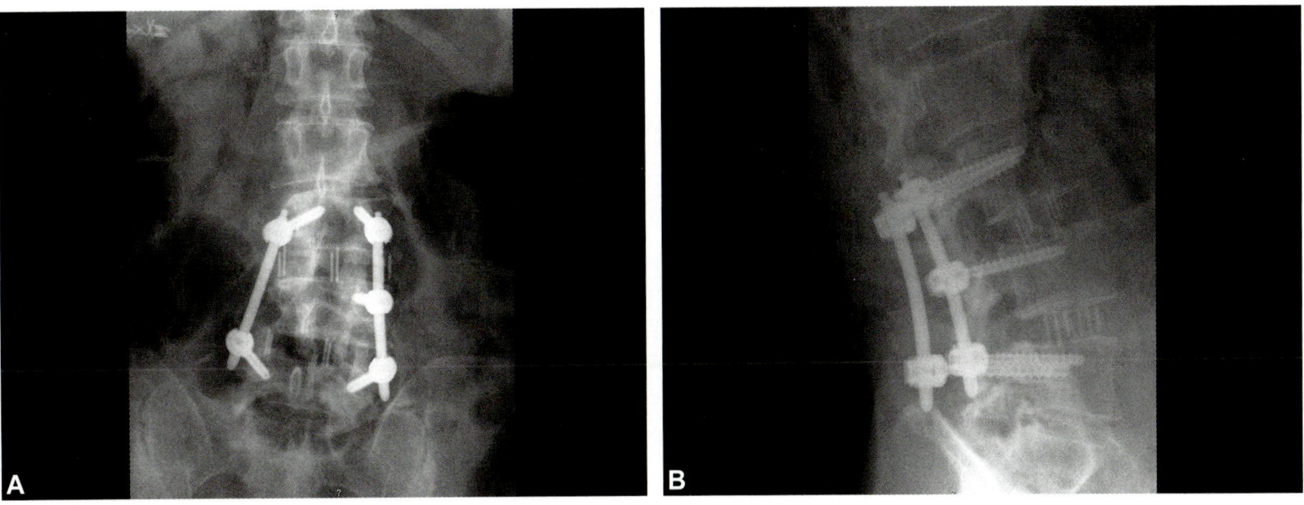

Figs. 10.13A and B: Final (A) anteroposterior and (B) lateral radiographs demonstrating appropriate position of the intervertebral cages.

POSTOPERATIVE CARE

Complications[2]

- Iliopsoas weakness
  - Most common complication (~22%)
  - Symptoms are typically transient with return to baseline after 2–6 weeks and no long-term sequelae.
  - Patients can benefit from physical and occupational therapy.
- Anterior thigh numbness (~18%)
  - Symptoms may last up to 12 months.
  - Patients may experience a partial or total return of sensation after 3–6 months.
- Quadriceps weakness (~7%) and foot drop (~2%)
  - There is a greater risk for lumbar plexus injury (i.e. femoral nerve injury) at the L4–L5 level due to the anterior trajectory of these nerve structures within the psoas muscles.
  - The resulting weakness may require physical therapy.
  - In cases of refractory weakness, the patients can develop quadriceps muscles atrophy.
- Radiculopathy (~7%)
  - New or worsening motor and sensory deficits can be noted post-operatively in a dermatomal distribution.
  - The initial management can range from observation to local nerve root steroid injection.
    - In general, symptoms are transient and resolve in 3–6 months.
- Peritoneal perforation (~2%)
  - Small lateral peritoneal perforations rarely require primary repair.

Complication Pearls

- Neurologic complications occur more often at the lower lumbar levels (L3–L4, L4–L5) due to a decreasing diameter of the safe working zone.
- Excessive or prolonged deployment of the retractor within the psoas muscle increases the risk of nerve injury.

- Vascular perforation (~2%)
  - If noted intraoperatively, the injured vessel can be repaired with endovascular clips.
  - Postoperative abdominal pain should warrant further imaging to rule out a retroperitoneal hematoma.
    - Angiography and embolization can be an effective treatment option.

EXPECTED AND ADVERSE OUTCOMES

- A direct lateral approach for an interbody fusion has a significantly reduced risk of injury to the great vessels when compared with the direct anterior approach.[3]
- A minimally invasive direct lateral approach to the lumbar spine is an effective procedure to correct coronal and sagittal plane deformities.[4]
- The transpsoas approach is associated with a 6.2–52% risk of neurologic complications related to the injury of the lumbar plexus.[2] A thorough knowledge of the patient anatomy and meticulous surgical technique can help prevent this cumbersome complication.[5]

REFERENCES

1. Uribe JS, Vale FL, Dakwar E. Electromyographic monitoring and its anatomical implications in minimally invasive spine surgery. Spine. 2010;35:S368-74.
2. Sofianos DA, Briseno MR, Abrams J, Patel AA. Complications of the lateral transpsoas approach for lumbar interbody arthrodesis: a case series and literature review. Clin Orthop Relat Res. 2012;470:1621-32.
3. Arnold PM, Anderson KK, McGuire RA, Jr. The lateral transpsoas approach to the lumbar and thoracic spine: A review. Surg Neurol Int. 2012;3:S198-215.
4. Phillips FM, Isaacs RE, Rodgers WB, et al. Adult degenerative scoliosis treated with XLIF: clinical and radiographic results of a prospective multi-center study with 24-month follow-up. Spine (Phila Pa 1976). 2013;38(21):1853-61.
5. Park DK, Lee MJ, Lin EL, et al. The relationship of intrapsoas nerves during a transpsoas approach to the lumbar spine anatomic study. J Spinal Disord Tech. 2010;23:223-8.

REFERENCE SUMMARY

1. Uribe JS, Vale FL, Dakwar E. Electromyographic monitoring and its anatomical implications in minimally invasive spine surgery. Spine. 2010;35:S368-74.
   Summary: A literature review on the different neuromonitoring methods utilized in minimally invasive spine surgery and its application in a lateral transpsoas approach. The authors conclude that neuromonitoring is crucial for the safe trajectory instruments through the psoas muscles during a minimally invasive lateral retroperitoneal approach.
2. Sofianos DA, Briseno MR, Abrams J, Patel AA. Complications of the lateral transpsoas approach for lumbar interbody arthrodesis: a case series and literature review. Clin OrthopRelat Res 2012;470:1621-32.
   Summary: A retrospective review of the complications incurred by 45 patients who underwent a retroperitoneal transpsoas approach for a lumbar interbody fusion. The authors reported a 40% incidence of postoperative neurological complications including iliopsoas weakness, quadriceps weakness, foot drop, and anterior thigh hypoesthesia.

3. Arnold PM, Anderson KK, McGuire RA, Jr. The lateral transpsoas approach to the lumbar and thoracic spine: A review. Surgical Neurology International 2012;3:S198-215.
Summary: A literature review comparing the different approaches for an interbody fusion in the thoracic and lumbar spine to the extreme lateral transpsoas approach (XLIF). The authors discuss, clinical indications, relevant anatomy, utilization of bone morphogenetic protein, complications, fusion rates, and clinical outcomes after an XLIF. The authors conclude that an XLIF is as cost-effective as other standard interbody fusion procedures.
4. Phillips FM, Isaacs RE, Rodgers WB, et al. Adult degenerative scoliosis treated with XLIF: clinical and radiographic results of a prospective multi-center study with 24-month follow-up. Spine (Phila Pa 1976) 2013;38(21):1853-61.
Summary: A prospective, multicenter analysis of the clinical and radiographic outcomes of 107 patients who underwent an extreme lateral interbody fusion (XLIF) for degenerative scoliosis. The authors reported significant improvement in clinical outcomes and radiographic correction of the spinal deformity at 24 months after the procedure.
5. Park DK, Lee MJ, Lin EL, Singh K, An HS, Phillips FM. The relationship of intrapsoas nerves during a transpsoas approach to the lumbar spine anatomic study. J Spinal Disord Tech 2010;23:223-8.
Summary: A cadaveric study to evaluate the relationship of the lumbar exiting nerve root and trunks within the psoas muscle with reference to the radiographic center of the intervertebral disc. The authors concluded that although, in most cases, the nerve structures are at a safe distance from the intervertebral disc center, neuromonitoring should be implemented during a direct lateral interbody fusion to account for anatomical variation and prevent injury.

Chapter

11

Mini-Open Anterior Lumbar Interbody Fusion

Alejandro Marquez-Lara, Branko Skovrlj, Sheeraz A Qureshi, Kern Singh

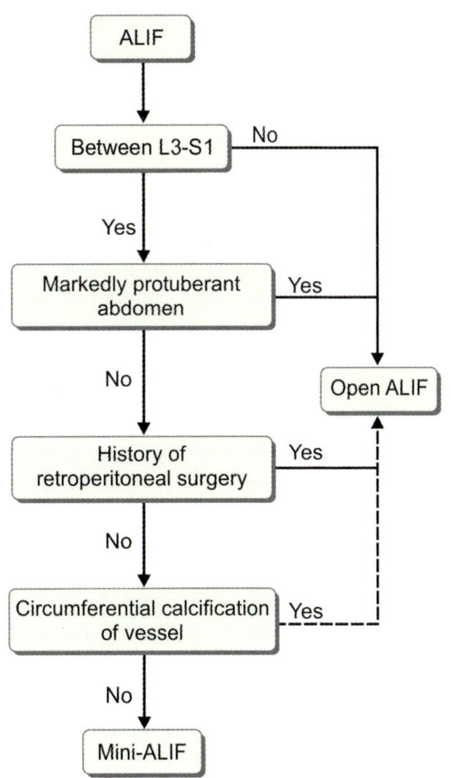

CASE VIGNETTE

A 67-year-old man presents to the office with a history of back and lower extremity pain that radiates into the plantar aspect of his left foot. On examination, the patient demonstrates weakness with plantar flexion and a diminished Achilles tendon reflex. The lumbar magnetic resonance imaging (MRI) demonstrates disc space collapse at L5–S1 with foraminal and lateral recess stenosis. The patient has failed 6 weeks of conservative therapy with physical therapy and anti-inflammatory and pain medications.

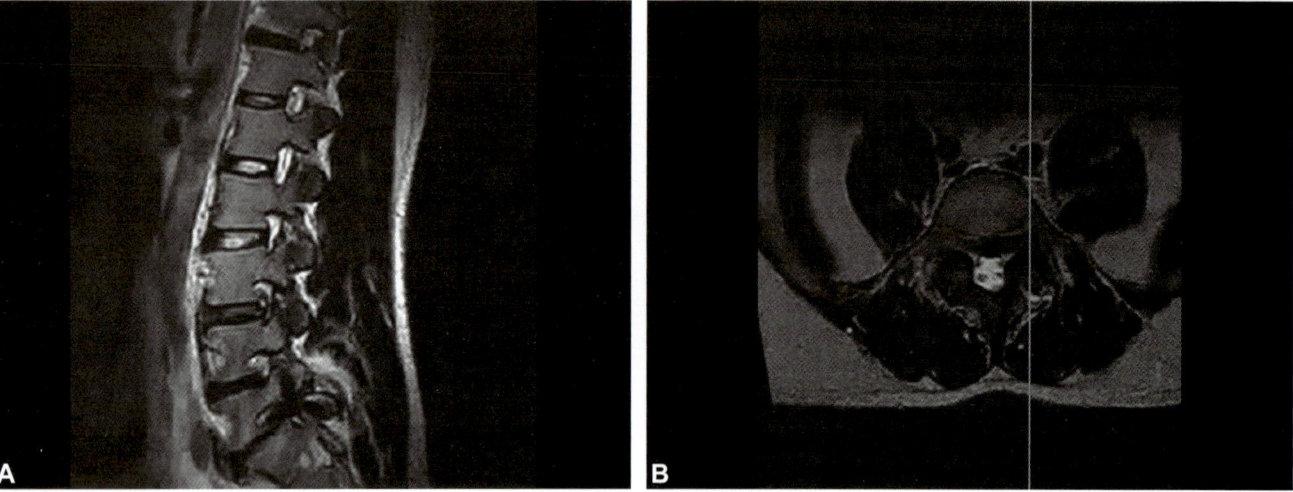

Figs. 11.1A and B: Preoperative (A) sagittal and (B) axial magnetic resonance image of the lumbar spine demonstrating an isthmic spondylolisthesis and left foraminal stenosis at L5–S1.

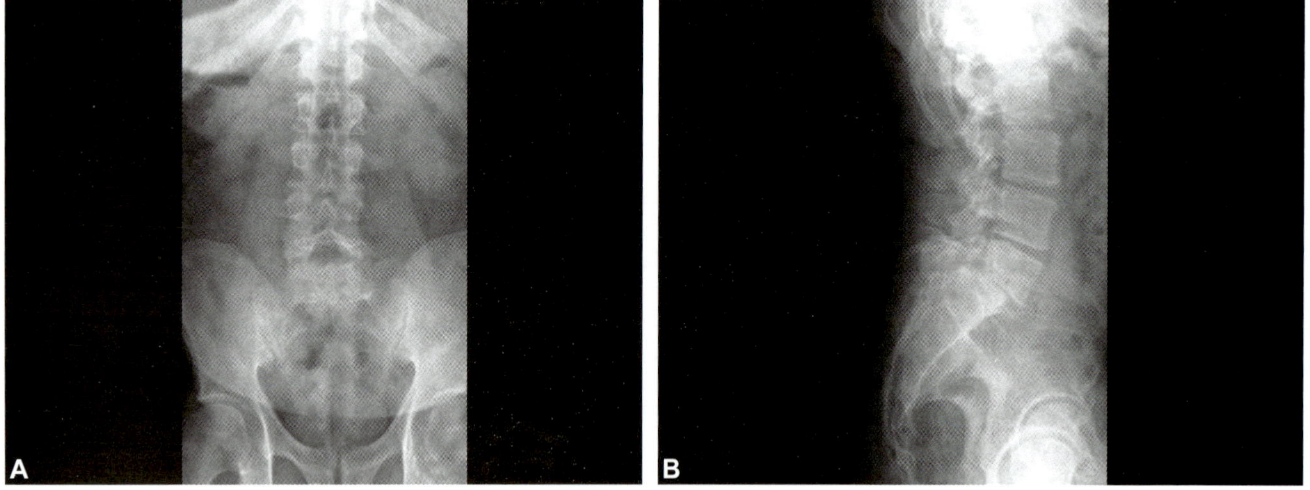

Figs. 11.2A and B: Preoperative (A) anteroposterior and (B) lateral radiograph demonstrating grade I–II spondylolisthesis at L5–S1.

DIAGNOSTIC IMAGING

- MRI (Figs. 11.1A and B)
  - MRI is the imaging modality of choice to identify and characterize the level and extent of the pathology.
  - Allows the surgeon to determine a safe approach by identifying critical structures including the great vessels and the lumbar plexus relative to the affected disc space
  - MRI should be evaluated for degeneration, endplate changes, annular tears, Modic changes, and high-intensity zones.
- Plain film radiograph—Anteroposterior (AP) and lateral (Figs. 11.2A and B).
  - Upright plain AP and lateral radiographs including flexion and extension views may be utilized to evaluate the overall coronal and sagittal alignment.

Imaging Pearls/Pitfalls

- On the standing lateral radiograph, the pubis should be evaluated to determine if visualization of the L5-S1 disc space will be compromised.

- Standing lateral lumbar radiographs should be utilized to assess the sacral slope and the L5–S1 disc to determine if the angle will allow for an anterior access.
- Radiographs should also be evaluated for degenerative changes including osteophyte formation, disc space narrowing, foraminal narrowing, vacuum phenomenon within the disc, and endplate sclerosis.
- Computed tomography (CT)
  - If an MRI is contraindicated (ocular implants, cardiac pacemakers, etc.), a CT myelogram can be utilized to investigate for spinal stenosis.
- Discography
  - Involves direct stimulation of the pathologic disc and is utilized in conjunction with MRI for suspected discogenic pathology

Surgical Indications

- Spinal instability
  - Degenerative disc disease
  - Spondylolisthesis
  - Postlaminectomy syndrome
  - Adjacent segment degeneration
  - Pseudarthrosis
  - Tumor
  - Infection

INSTRUMENTATION

- Radiolucent surgical table
- Intraoperative fluoroscopy
- Surgical loupes
- Expandable retractor and table-mounted retractor arm
- Intervertebral disc spacers or cages
- Bone graft or bone graft substitutes
- Shavers
- Curettes
- Rasps
- Cobb elevators

POSITIONING AND INTRAOPERATIVE SETUP

- The patient should be placed into a supine position (Fig. 11.3).
- The break of the surgical bed is positioned at either the top of the iliac crest or higher depending upon the lumbar level of operation (L3–L4 to L5–S1). Lowering the top end of the bed will open the disc space.
  - A lumbar bolster can accentuate lordosis if needed.
- The arms are folded and secured over the chest while ensuring appropriate padding of the elbows and between the hands. This allows the C-arm to be prepped into the surgical field in a lateral position.
- The fluoroscopy monitor should be on the opposite side of the surgeon.

Indication Pearls

- An anterior approach greatly reduces the potential injury to the dura mater and the neural elements.
- With a miniopen anterior lumbar interbody fusion (ALIF), the peritoneum is not entered. This leads to a better visualization of the intra-abdominal vessels, faster recovery (lack of ileus), and a limited potential for visceral complications.

Contraindications/Pitfalls

- Calcification of the vessels (evaluated by CT)
- Obesity
- History of retroperitoneal surgery (scars and altered landmarks)
- High pelvic brim limiting visualization of the disc space
- Males have a 2–5% risk for retrograde ejaculation with an anterior approach.

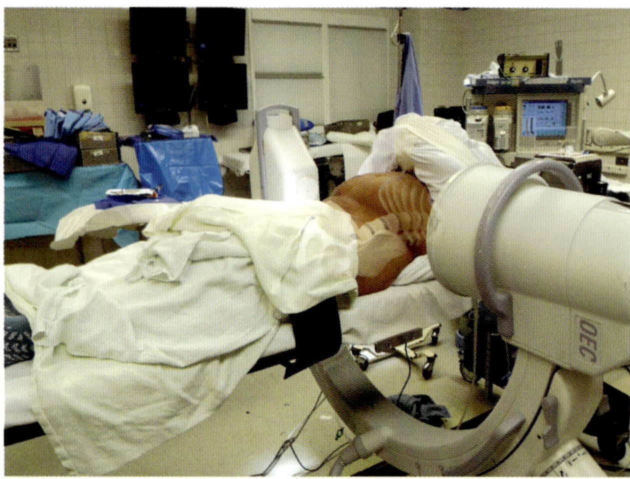

Fig. 11.3: The patient is placed in a supine position with the arms tucked and secured over the chest.

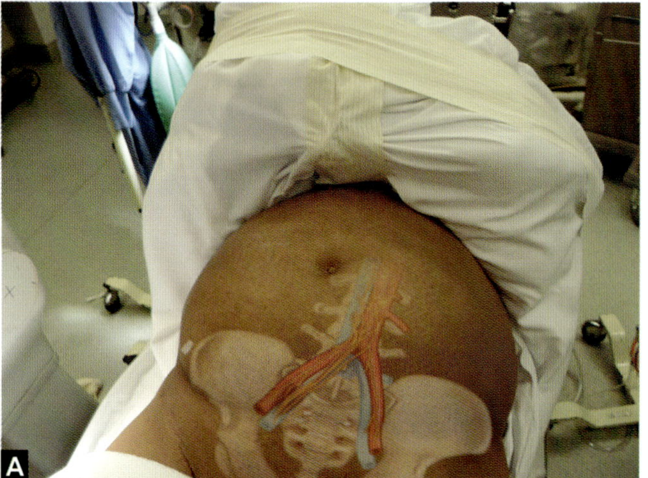

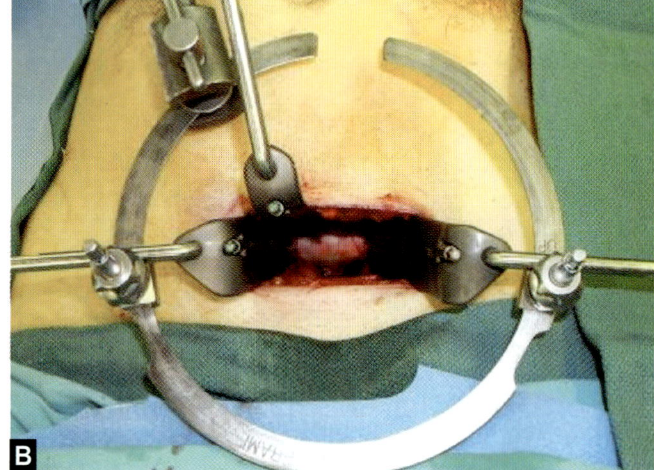

Figs. 11.4A and B: Intraoperative view of (A) the incision site and (B) retractor system utilized in the mini-anterior lumbar interbody fusion approach.

SURGICAL ANATOMY AND EXPOSURE

Relevant Anatomy (Figs. 11.4A and B)

At the L5–S1 level, the great vessels (aorta/vena cava) have bifurcated. At L4–L5, the great vessels are retracted to the right and the ascending lumbar vein is ligated to mobilize the vessels. The anterior approach poses a significant risk to the ureter, sympathetic nerves, and the hypogastric plexus.

Surgical Exposure

- A transverse incision is made at the level of the iliac crest for single level surgery at L4–L5 or slightly below the iliac crest for L5–S1 (Fig. 11.5). Confirmation prior to the incision via fluoroscopic imaging is essential to center the incision and to minimize the dissection.
  - For multilevel procedures, a vertical incision may be utilized.

Exposure Pearls

- At L4–L5, care must be taken to identify the ascending lumbar vein. In addition, care must be taken to prevent excessive traction on the vein while retracting the great vessels to the right.
- Hand-held retractors may be used because the fatigue factor of the assistant will allow intermittent blood flow during the course of the procedure.
- Care should be taken to identify the ureter. The ureter should be retracted with the retroperitoneal contents.
- Avoidance of electrocautery may reduce the risk of retrograde ejaculation. Alternatively, a bipolar cautery can be utilized to achieve hemostasis.

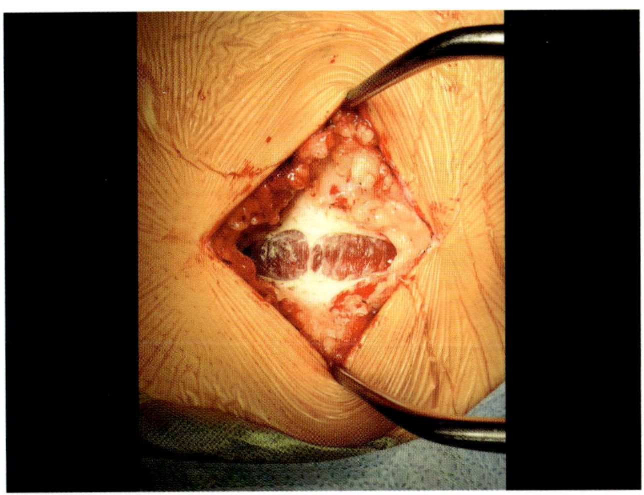

Fig. 11.5: Intraoperative photograph demonstrating the rectus muscle fibers.

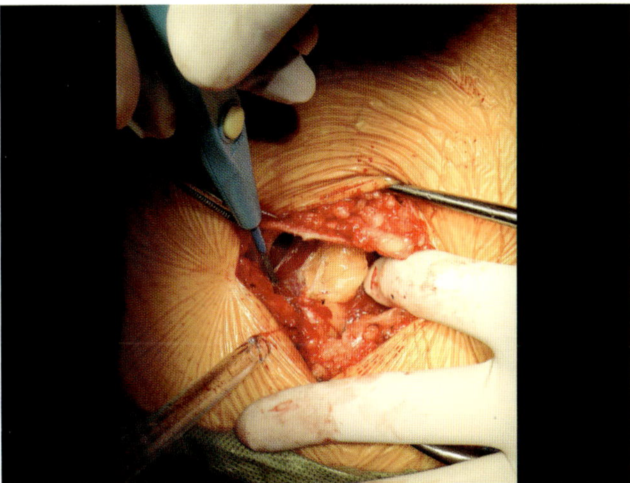

Fig. 11.6: Intraoperative photograph demonstrating dissection under the left rectus muscle.

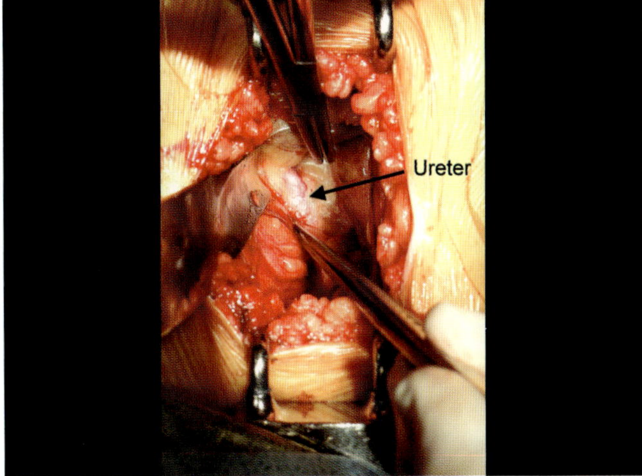

Fig. 11.7: Intraoperative view of the surgical field identifying the ureter. The anatomic structures encountered with this approach are meticulously identified and carefully retracted to expose the disc space.

- After the skin and subcutaneous tissues are divided, the anterior rectus sheath is identified and split transversely. Some surgeons prefer a vertical fascial incision particularly for multilevel exposures.
- A surgical plane is created underneath the left rectus (Fig. 11.6). The transversalis fascia is identified and separated from the underlying peritoneum, which is dissected laterally.
- Carefully, the peritoneum is dissected around the abdominal wall over the psoas.
- If the ascending lumbar vein does not need to be resected, the vessels are carefully mobilized to the right until the disc space is adequately exposed (Fig. 11.7).
- For the L5-S1 level, the peritoneum and the presacral nerves should be elevated in one clean plane to prevent retrograde ejaculation.

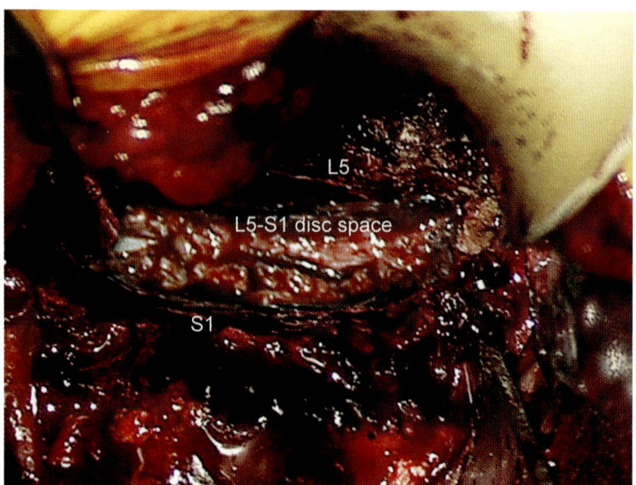

Fig. 11.8: Direct visualization of the target disc space prior to the annulotomy.

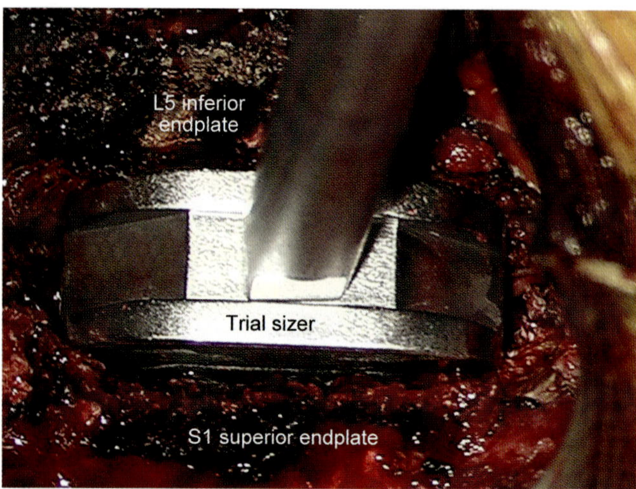

Fig. 11.9: A trial sizer is inserted in the intervertebral disc space after completing the discectomy and preparing the endplates.

Procedure-specific Steps

- Step 1
  - Once the left and right common iliac arteries and veins are retracted, the disc space is identified.
- Step 2
  - An annulotomy is performed with either a knife or an electrocautery device. This procedure is similar to the endplate preparation performed during an anterior cervical discectomy and fusion (Fig. 11.8).
- Step 3
  - A ring curette is utilized after incising the annulus. The annulus is then detached from the endplate with a Cobb elevator. As much disc as possible should be removed; however, care must be taken not to injure the endplates during the discectomy as this predisposes to subsequent implant migration and subsidence.
- Step 4
  - The disc space is distracted to match the height of the normal adjacent vertebrae and disc space.
- Step 5
  - A sizing device should be utilized to assess the appropriate size of the cage or graft (Fig. 11.9).
  - Again, care must be taken not to damage the vertebral endplates during this stage.
- Step 6
  - The appropriately sized implant is packed with graft material and placed into the disc space.
  - The implant will restore the size of the intervertebral space, indirectly increasing the caliber of the vertebral foramina.
  - Insertion of a tapered device will also restore lumbar spinal lordosis.

Procedural Pearls/Pitfalls

- During the annulotomy, the blade edge should be pointed away from the vascular structures.
- Perforation to the endplates may increase the likelihood of implant subsidence and migration.
- Incomplete discectomy can result in the retropulsion of disc fragments into the spinal canal when the implant is positioned.
- A lateral and posteriorly placed implant can cause neuroforaminal impingement.

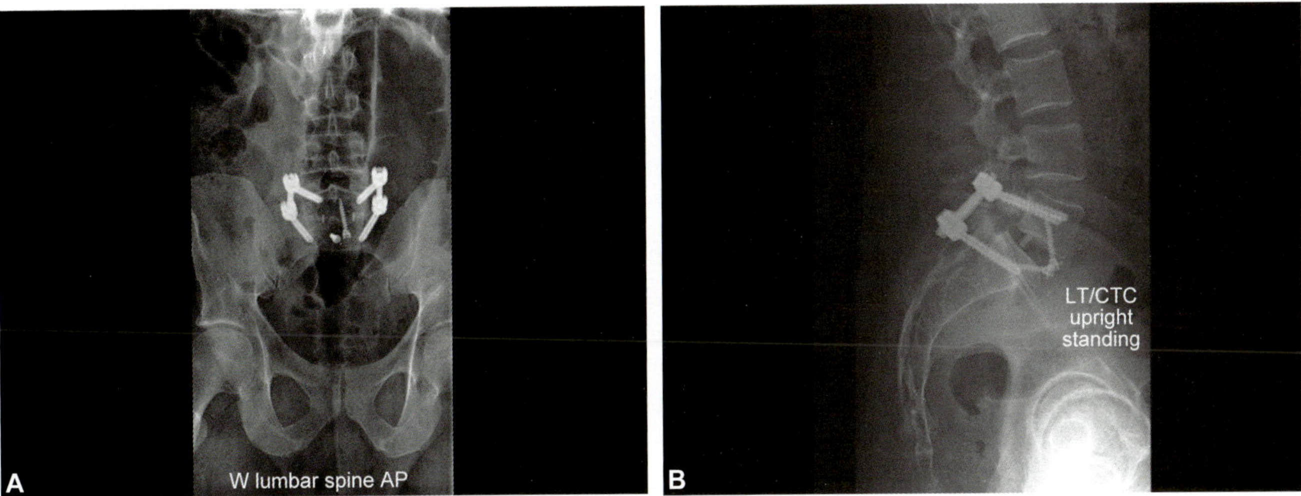

Figs. 11.10A and B: Postoperative (A) anteroposterior and (B) lateral radiograph demonstrating the final construct after anterior lumbar interbody fusion with interbody cage and posterior percutaneous pedicle fixation.

- Step 7
    - Lateral fluoroscopy should be obtained to ensure correct placement of the implant.
    - AP image should also be obtained to confirm that the implant is centered within the disc space (Figs. 11.10A and B).

POSTOPERATIVE CARE

Adverse Outcomes

- Peritoneal perforation
    - If the peritoneal perforation is small and lateral, a primary repair is infrequently required.
    - If the perforation is ventral, a formal repair should be performed to avoid a postoperative hernia.
- Vessel injury
    - The reported vascular injury rate is 1.9%.[2]
    - If a vascular repair is warranted, clips are the most effective means of repairing venous tears, but occasionally sutures can be utilized. An arterial injury rarely occurs.
- Vessel thrombosis
    - Thrombosis of the artery or vein is rare.
    - Intraoperative monitoring utilizing an oximeter on the toes of the left foot should be utilized because the left side is most often occluded.
    - Intermittent relaxation of the retractors will allow blood flow to occur.
- Ureter injury
    - Injury to the ureter is very rare; it can be identified immediately or may present postoperatively as a urinoma.

Procedural Pearls/Pitfalls

- An angled insertion of the implant will fracture the subchondral bone resulting in a loss of lordosis and implant subsidence.
- Poor bone quality and bone healing may potentiate a symptomatic pseudarthrosis.
- A small implant size and poor annular tension can result in dislodgment, pseudarthrosis, and subsidence.
- The improper closure of the fascial layers can result in a direct hernia.
- A lateral peritoneal perforation may not require a repair. In contrast, a ventral perforation will require repair to reduce the risk for herniation.
- Clips are the most effective means to repair vein tears but occasionally sutures are utilized.

- Sympathetic effect
  - Patients may complain of a cold leg on the contralateral side of the procedure because the approach side will have greater blood flow. These sympathetically-mediated symptoms should resolve within 2–3 months.
- Lymphatic injury
  - A very rare complication typically treated conservatively
  - The surgeon may notice chyle regressing from the injured lymphatics.
  - The lymphatics can be repaired by utilizing clips. Rarely, a drain may be necessary.
- Nerve root injury
  - The surgeon must be mindful with the lateral dissection and with the placement of the retractors.
  - The L5 nerve root may be compressed if the retractors are positioned too deep on the right side with a left-sided approach at the L5–S1 level.
- Injury to the presacral parasympathetic plexus
  - Injury to the nerve plexus may result in retrograde ejaculation in males.[3]
  - The risk is minimized with a miniopen approach because the peritoneum is dissected off the anterior aspect of the spine at L5–S1, and the nerves are retracted with the peritoneum.[4]
- Abdominal visceral injury
  - If electrocautery is utilized to cut the last layer of the fascia or the transversalis fascia, care must be taken to prevent perforation of the peritoneum.
  - This complication should be managed with the approach surgeon.[5]

Adverse Outcomes Pearls/Pitfalls

- An access surgeon can be utilized for the exposure depending upon the level of experience of the spine surgeon.
- Compression of the left iliac vessels by the retractors can cause distal desaturation, which has been correlated with SSEP changes seen after the placement and removal of the retractors.[1]
- A pulse oximeter can be placed on the left great toe to indirectly measure perfusion to the extremity.
- Placement of the retractor is paramount to prevent nerve root injury.
- The risk of vascular complications may be reduced by checking a preoperative CT for calcification of the vessels.

REFERENCES

1. Brau SA, Spoonamore MJ, Snyder L, et al. Nerve monitoring changes related to iliac artery compression during anterior lumbar spine surgery. Spine J. 2003;3:351-5.
2. Brau SA, Delamarter RB, Schiffman ML, et al. Vascular injury during anterior lumbar surgery. Spine J. 2004;4:409-12.
3. Burkus JK, Dryer RF, Peloza JH. Retrograde ejaculation following single-level anterior lumbar surgery with or without recombinant human bone morphogenetic protein-2 in 5 randomized controlled trials: clinical article. J Neuros Spine. 2013;18:112-21.
4. Kaiser MG, Haid RW, Jr, Subach BR, et al. Comparison of the mini-open versus laparoscopic approach for anterior lumbar interbody fusion: a retrospective review. Neurosurgery. 2002;51:97-103.
5. Brau SA. Mini-open approach to the spine for anterior lumbar interbody fusion: description of the procedure, results and complications. Spine J. 2002;2:216-23.

REFERENCE SUMMARY

4. Kaiser MG, Haid RW, Jr., Subach BR, et al. Comparison of the mini-open versus laparoscopic approach for anterior lumbar interbody fusion: a retrospective review. Neurosurgery 2002;51:97-103.
Summary: The mini-open and the laparoscopic techniques are both effective ALIF procedures. The laparoscopic technique did not demonstrate superiority over the mini-open laparotomy. The authors concluded that the mini-open ALIF approach is preferred due to its theoretical advantages including the direct access to the disc interspace, complete disc removal, resection of herniated fragments, an increased endplate exposure, and a significnalty reduced incidence of a mini-open laparotomy.
5. Brau SA. Mini-open approach to the spine for anterior lumbar interbody fusion: description of the procedure, results and complications. Spine J. 2002; 2:216-23.
Summary: This article provides a technical description of the miniopen ALIF. The reported 6-month complications include arterial injury (0.8%), venous injury (0.8%), DVT (1.0%), ileus (0.6%), and infection (0.4%). The author concluded that the miniopen approach is safe and effective but is associated with a significant learning curve.

Chapter

12

Axial Lumbar Interbody Fusion

Sreeharsha V Nandyala, Rahul Kamath, Kern Singh

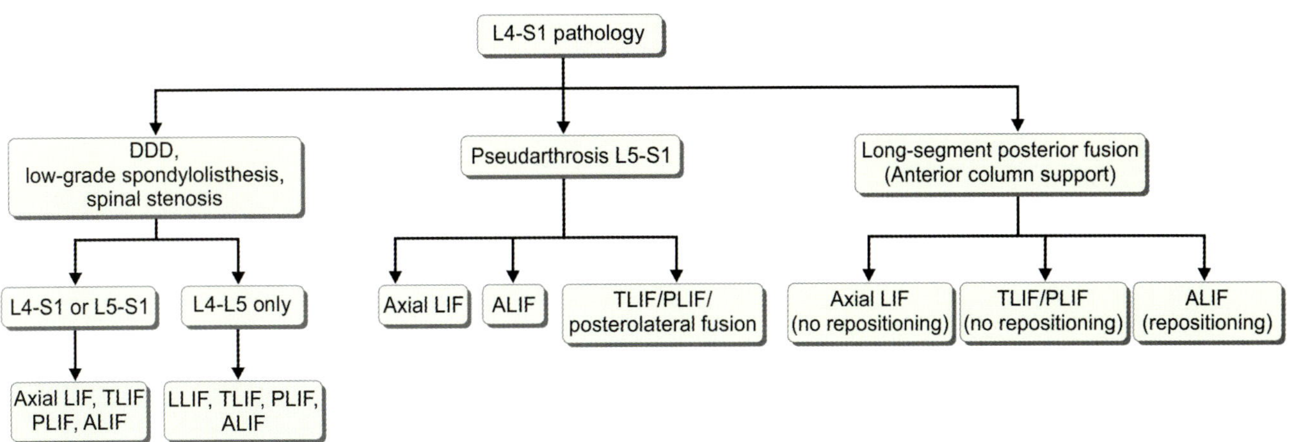

CASE VIGNETTE

A 59-year-old man presents to the office with back and leg pain. The patient describes a long history of back pain, but with new onset right lower extremity numbness, tingling, and pain. On examination, he demonstrates diminished sensation on the lateral aspect of his right foot as well as plantar flexion weakness when compared with the left side. Imaging studies demonstrate a degenerative L5–S1 spondylolisthesis and spinal stenosis. Conservative management with nonsteroidal medication, physical therapy, and epidural injections offered minimal symptom relief.

DIAGNOSTIC IMAGING

Plain Film Radiograph—Anteroposterior (AP), Lateral, and Full Sacral Views (Fig. 12.1)

- Adequate imaging enables initial evaluation of the bony anatomy to help determine if the patient is suitable for this surgical technique.

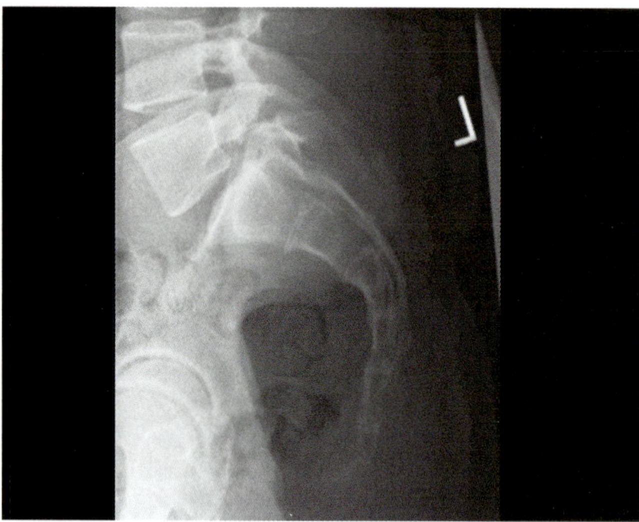

Fig. 12.1: Preoperative lateral radiograph demonstrating L5–S1 grade I isthmic spondylolisthesis. The entire length of the sacrum is included to aid in the preoperative planning.

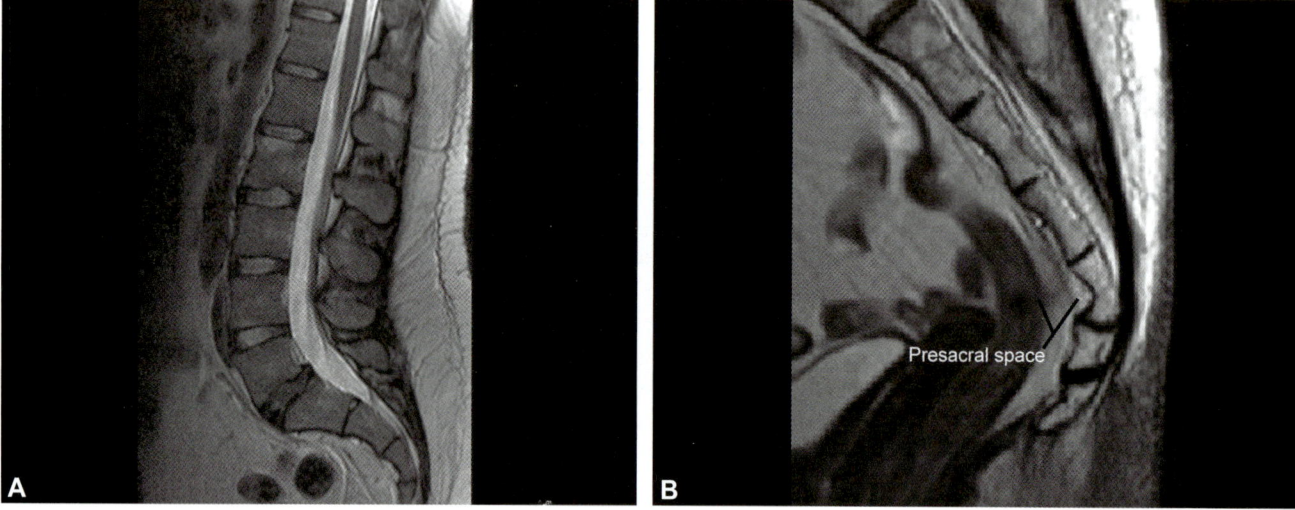

Figs. 12.2A and B: Preoperative (A) sagittal magnetic resonance image (MRI) demonstrating L5–S1 grade I spondylolisthesis. (B) The width of the presacral space is measured on a midsagittal MRI.

Magnetic Resonance Imaging (MRI) (Fig. 12.2A)

- It is essential for the MRI to include the tip of the coccyx to evaluate the presacral space (Fig. 12.2B).
  - On a midsagittal MRI the presacral space is bordered anteriorly by the visceral peritoneum of the rectum and posteriorly by the presacral fascia.
  - The presacral space should be evaluated for the perirectal fat pad thickness and anomalous vascular anatomy.
    - These findings will help delineate the rectal-sacrum interface.
- Careful assessment of the MRI imaging is critical to ensure feasibility and safety of the planned procedure.
  - Preoperative templating (Fig. 12.3)

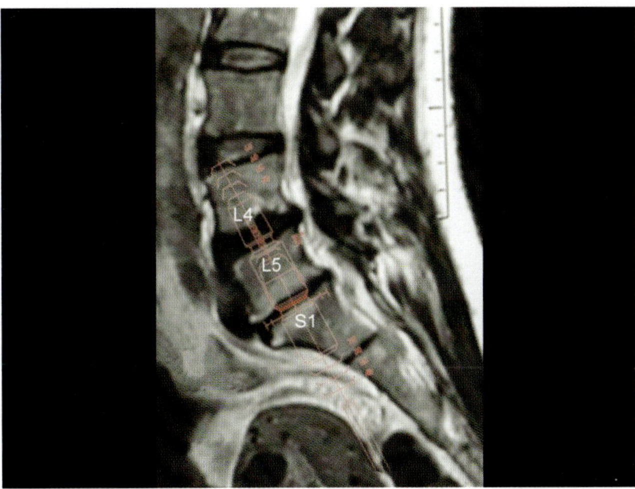

Fig. 12.3: A preoperative midsagittal magnetic resonance image is utilized to determine the trajectory and size of the implant.

- On a sagittal MRI, a line is drawn from the entry point below the sacrococcygeal joint to the midpoint of the S1 endplate.
  - The optimal trajectory of the implant is perpendicular to the superior S1 endplate.
- The implant template should fit leaving >6 mm from both the anterior and posterior walls of the L4 and L5 bodies and at least 7 mm from the posterior border of S1.
- Lastly, the implant should clear the posterior rectal wall and peritoneum on the sagittal plane.

SURGICAL INDICATIONS

- L4–S1 pathology
  - Degenerative disc disease
  - Spinal stenosis
  - Pseudarthrosis (previous failed fusions)
  - Spondylolisthesis (Grades I and II)
  - Postlaminectomy instability
  - Degenerative scoliosis

Indication Pearls

- Axial LIF can be utilized in deformity cases to restore disc height and lumbar lordosis.
- Significant lumbosacral coronal deformity should be corrected with posterior pedicle screws and rods prior to an axial fusion.

Contraindications/Pitfalls

- In patients with only L4–L5 pathology, an alternative fusion technique should be pursued [lateral lumbar interbody fusion (LLIF), transforaminal lumbar interbody fusion (TLIF), anterior lumbar interbody fusion (ALIF)].
- Contraindications include diverticulitis, inflammatory bowel disease, or previous pelvic surgery. These conditions may be associated with pelvic tissue scarring.

INSTRUMENTATION

- Radiolucent surgical table
- Intraoperative fluoroscopy (x2)
  - Lateral
  - AP
- Blunt cannula probe
- Drill
- Sheaths/cannula
- Guide pin
- Bone graft

- Nitinol disc cutters
- Tissue extractors
- Rod implants
  - L5–S1 nondistracting
  - L5–S1 distracting
    - Modular rod composed of an L5 anchor, S1 anchor, distraction rod, and fixation rod
- L4–S1 2-level distracting
  - Modular rod composed of an L4–L5 anchor, S1 anchor, distraction rod and fixation rod

POSITIONING AND INTRAOPERATIVE SETUP

- The patient is positioned prone on a Jackson table, and the bony prominences are appropriately padded.
  - Hip pads are placed to elevate the sacrum, allowing axial entry to the lumbosacral spine.
- The lower back and gluteal region are prepped and draped with standard sterile technique.
- The surgeon should be positioned such that his/her dominant arm is toward the feet, which will facilitate instrument manipulation.

Positioning Pearls

- Placement of a Foley catheter and insufflation in the rectum can help visualize the rectum (air) on fluoroscopy during the procedure.

SURGICAL ANATOMY AND EXPOSURE

Relevant Anatomy

- The presacral space is bordered anteriorly by the visceral peritoneum of the mesorectum and posteriorly by the presacral fascia overlying the venous plexus and sacrum.
- The presacral space is wider in males (16.2 mm at S-1 and 13.0 mm at S-3) than in females (11.9 mm at S-1 and 10.6 mm at S-3) in the sagittal plane. As such, women have a theoretically greater risk of rectal perforation, vascular injury, and damage to the presacral fascia.
- The middle sacral artery is usually small at the sacral promontory and is at minimal risk of injury during the approach.

Surgical Exposure

- A 2-cm paracoccygeal incision is made by palpating the paracoccygeal notch at the superior gluteal fold (Fig. 12.4).
- The parietal fascia is reached through blunt dissection and a blunt trocar is utilized to gain access into the presacral space (Fig. 12.5).
  - AP fluoroscopic imaging enables the surgeon to center the trocar on the anterior sacrum (Fig. 12.6).
- The lateral fluoroscopic image is then utilized to advance the trocar along the anterior sacrum until the tip reaches the level of the S1–S2 disc space.
- Trajectory of the trocar is then redirected toward the center of the L5–S1 disc space utilizing the lateral radiograph (Fig. 12.7).

Exposure Pearls

- A standard presurgical bowel preparation should be performed the night prior to surgery.
- Placing the guide pin at the correct starting point and proper trajectory is critical to assure adequate positioning of the rod across the vertebral bodies.

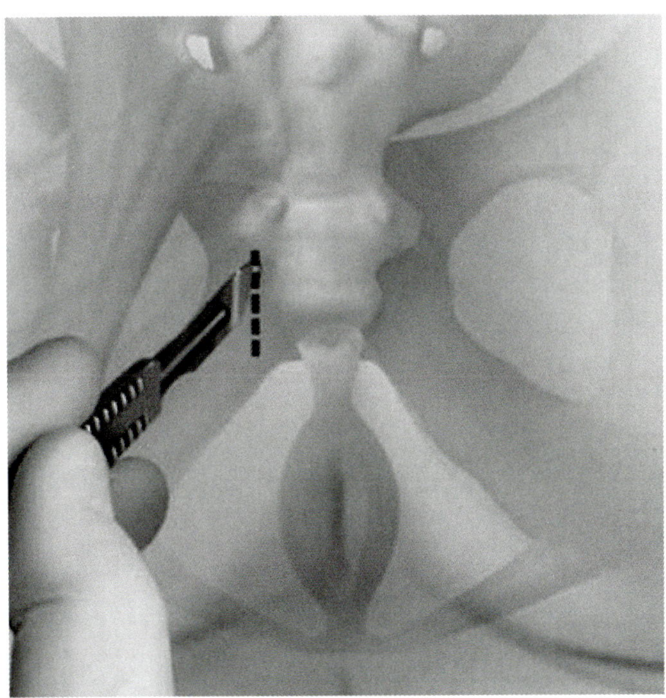

Fig. 12.4: Illustration demonstrating the site for the paracoccygeal incision.

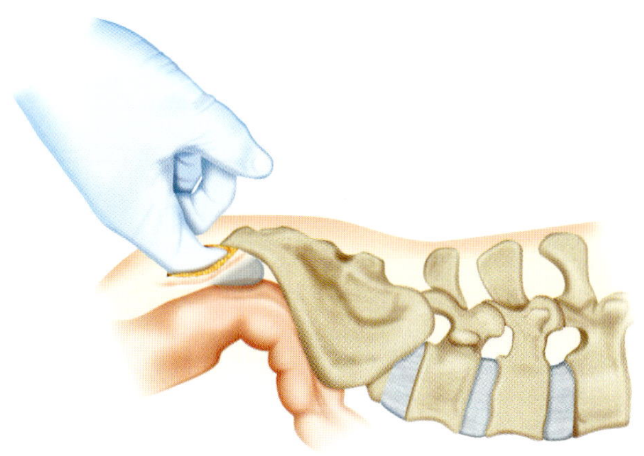

Fig. 12.5: Blunt dissection of the presacral space. The surgeon's finger palpates the tip of the coccyx posteriorly while mobilizing the rectum anteriorly.

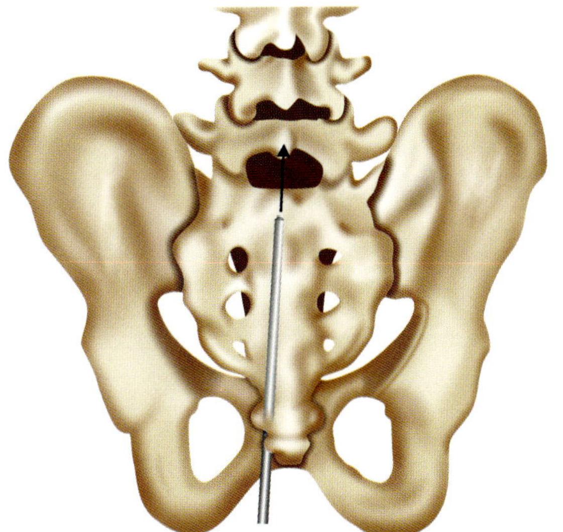

Fig. 12.6: On the anteroposterior plane, the trocar is centered on the anterior sacrum.

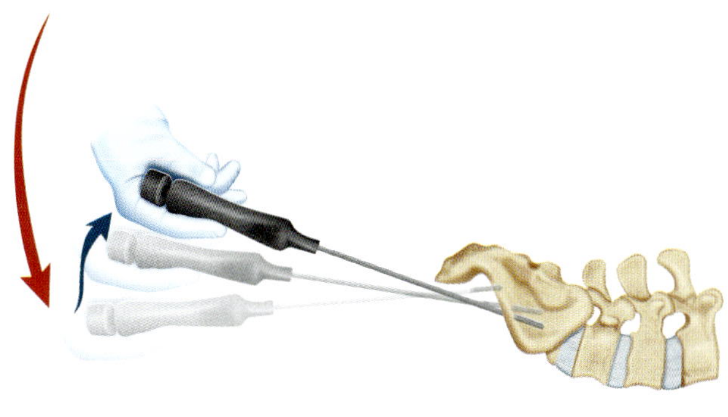

Fig. 12.7: The trocar is advanced along the anterior sacrum until reaching the starting point centered on the L5–S1 disc space.

- A guide pin is placed through the trocar and tapped into the sacrum. The trocar is removed, leaving the guide pin in place (Fig. 12.8).
- Sequential dilators are utilized to create a transosseous working channel into the sacrum and a 10-mm working sheath is left in place. The guide pin is then removed.

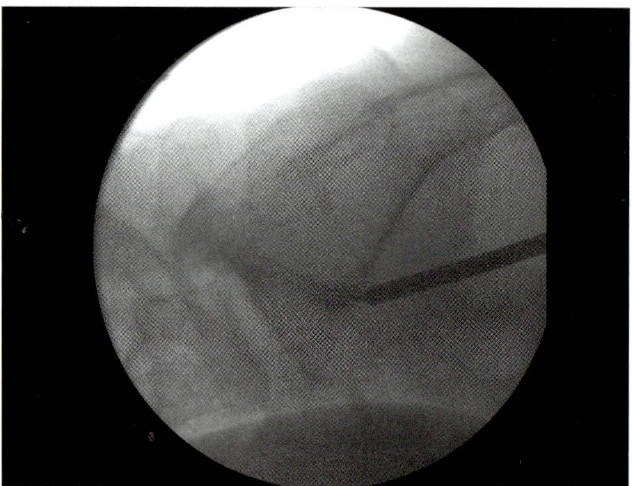

Fig. 12.8: Intraoperative lateral radiograph demonstrating the trajectory of the guide pin as it is inserted at the S1–S2 disc space and directed toward the center of the L5–S1 disc space.

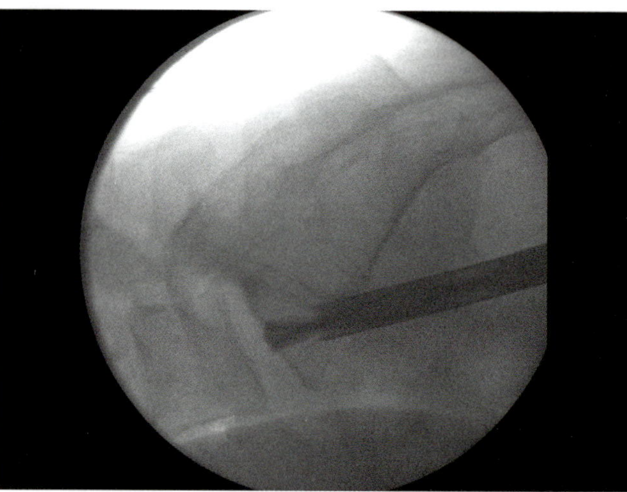

Fig. 12.9: A lateral radiograph depicting the use of a drill to expand the working channel into the L5–S1 disc space.

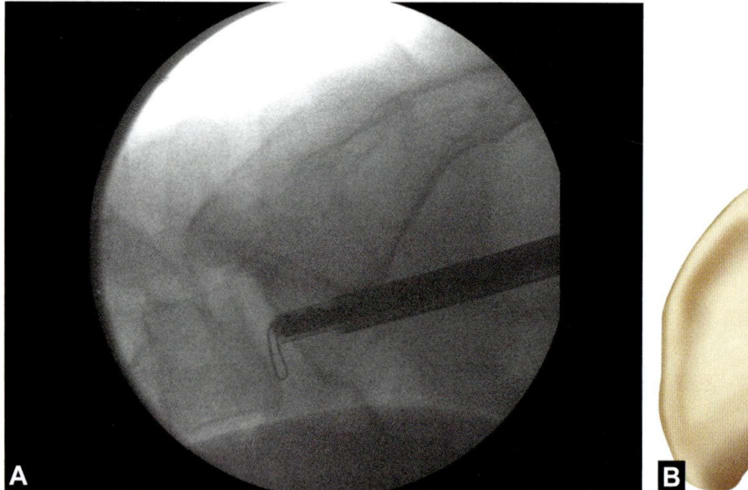

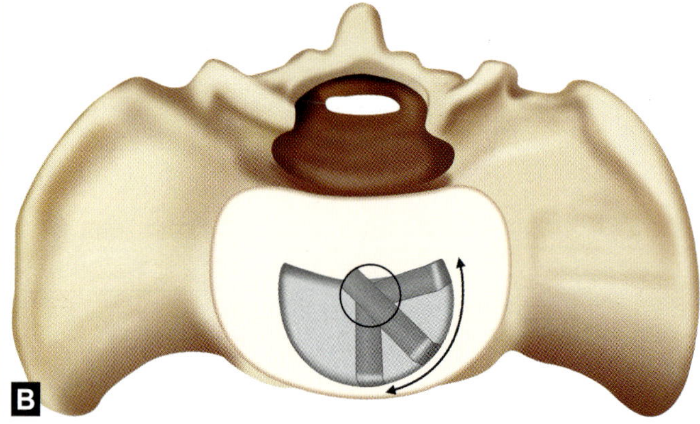

Figs. 12.10A and B: (A) Intraoperative lateral fluoroscopy demonstrating the disc cutter resecting the L5–S1 intervertebral disc. (B) Illustration of an axial view as the disc cutter removes the intervertebral disc.

PROCEDURE-SPECIFIC STEPS

- Step 1
  - Through the 10-mm sheath, a 9-mm drill is utilized to expand the working channel into the L5-S1 disc space (Fig. 12.9).
- Step 2
  - L5-S1 discectomy is performed with a series of nitinol disc cutters, which remove the nucleus pulposus and scrape the endplates leaving a bed of bleeding bone for fusion (Figs. 12.10A and B). The annulus fibrosus should be left intact.
- Step 3
  - The excised tissue is removed by tissue extractors, and the hollowed disc space is filled with bone graft.

Step 3 Pearls

- The tissue extractor should be utilized intermittently between the nitinol cutters to maintain the disc space clear of debris.

    - Autologous bone graft from local bone harvest, or a bone graft substitute can be utilized.
- Step 4

The remainder of the procedure depends upon the levels of fusion, as the implant size and dimensions will differ.

- L5-S1 nondistracting rod
    - The L5 body is drilled under lateral fluoroscopic guidance with a 7.5-mm drill and a measuring device (guide pin) is inserted to determine the length of the axial rod.
    - An exchange cannula is inserted to establish a working channel for implantation of the axial rod.
        - The exchange cannula should be positioned flush with the sacrum.
    - The nondistracting rod is inserted over the guidewire across the L5-S1 disc space under fluoroscopic guidance.
    - If necessary, a "material inserter" is introduced into the cannulated rod to deliver bone void filler. Lastly, a rod plug is then inserted to fill the axial rod.
- L5-S1 distracting rod
    - The 10-mm working channel in the sacrum is dilated with a 10.5-mm drill. A 12-mm sheath is then advanced through the sacrum until reaching the inferior endplate of L5.
    - The L5 vertebral body is then drilled with the 10.5-mm drill and a measuring device determines the implant size.
    - An exchange cannula is then inserted as above to create room for implant insertion.
    - The implant rod is advanced until the L5 anchor is completely engaged in the L5 vertebral body.
    - A counter torque tube is inserted followed by the distraction rod to restore the disc height.
    - Lastly, the fixation rod is inserted into the cannula to complete the construct (Figs. 12.11A to C).
- L4-S1 distracting rod
    - After gaining access to the inferior endplate of the L5 vertebra as above, the 10.5-mm drill is utilized to extend the working channel to the L4-L5 disc space.
    - Discectomy, endplate preparation, and bone graft placement is performed in the same fashion as the L5-S1 disc space (described above).
    - The L4 vertebra is then drilled with the 9-mm drill bit under lateral fluoroscopic guidance.
    - After determining the implant size with a trial rod, the assembled implant is inserted until the L4-L5 rod is engaged in the vertebra.
        - The S1 anchor should not cross the disc space into the L5 body.
    - The distraction rod is then advanced to distract the L5-S1 disc space.
    - Lastly, the fixation rod is inserted through the S1 anchor locking all of the components together (Fig. 12.12).

Procedure Pearls

- The L4-L5 rod has variable thread pitch and diameter that provides distraction of the L4-L5 disc space.
- Posterior stabilization with percutaneous posterior pedicle screw fixation is recommended to supplement the axial fusion.

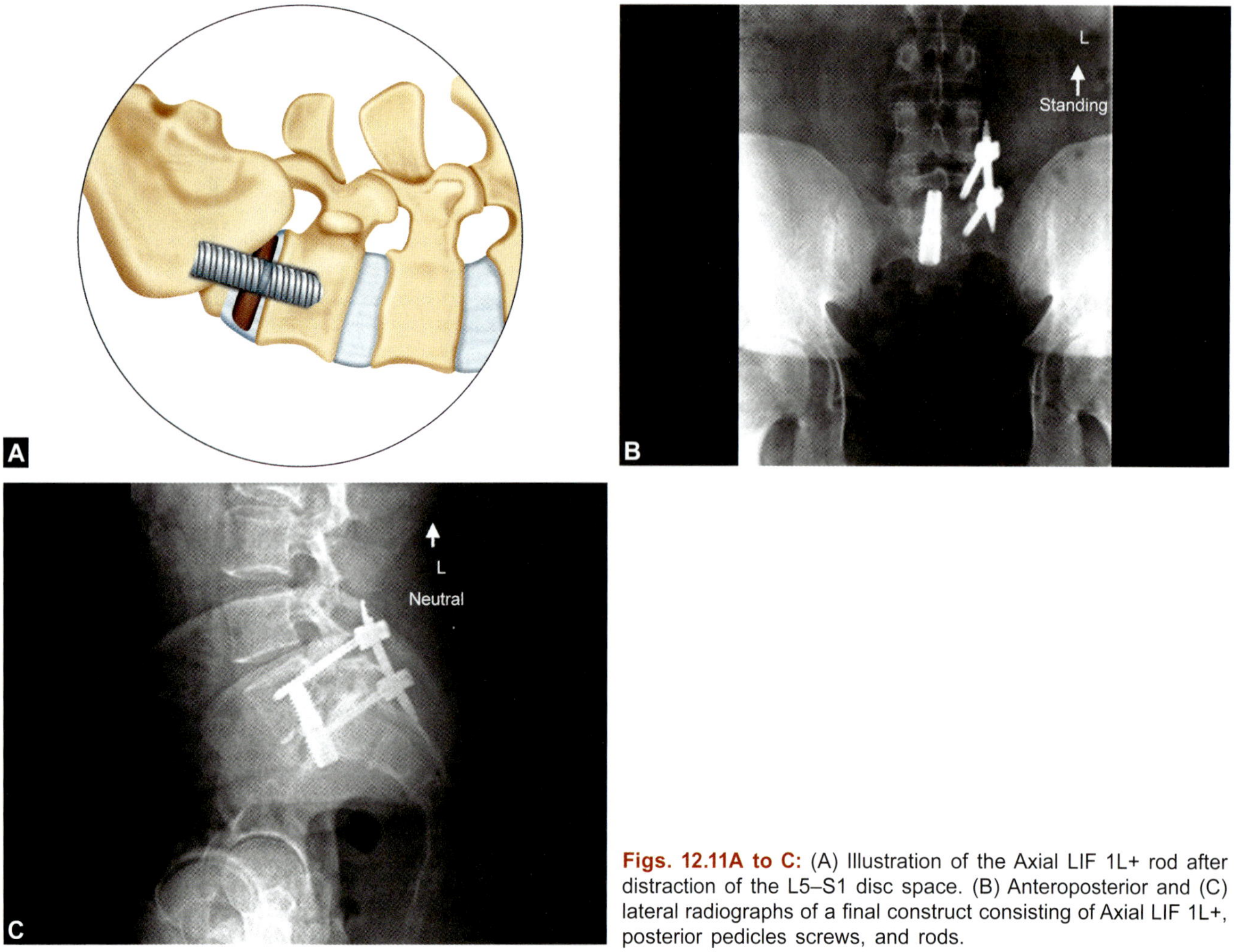

Figs. 12.11A to C: (A) Illustration of the Axial LIF 1L+ rod after distraction of the L5–S1 disc space. (B) Anteroposterior and (C) lateral radiographs of a final construct consisting of Axial LIF 1L+, posterior pedicles screws, and rods.

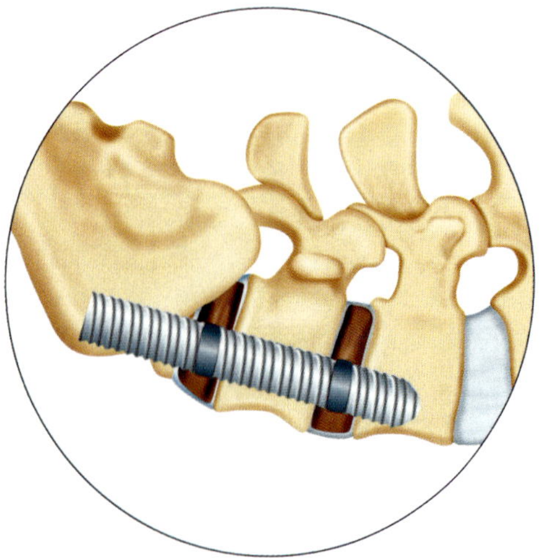

Fig. 12.12: Illustration of the Axial LIF 2L+ rod after distraction of the L4–L5 and L5–S1 disc spaces.

POSTOPERATIVE CARE

Adverse Outcomes

- Superficial wound infection (5.9%)
    - Superficial infections are often successfully treated conservatively with oral or IV antibiotics.
        - If necessary, a formal irrigation and drainage should be utilized.
- Pseudarthrosis (8.8%)
    - Patients who develop a pseudarthrosis can benefit from other fusion procedures including ALIF, posterior LIF (PLIF), or TLIF. Removing the axial rod through the potentially scarred presacral area may increase the risk of visceral injury. The anterior approach is a safe alternative for removal of the implant if indicated.
- Rectal perforation (0.6–2.9%)
    - This is the most important complication to avoid.
    - Careful preoperative history should be obtained. A history of diverticulitis, pelvic inflammatory disease, and previous pelvic procedures can significantly increase the risk of rectal injury.
    - Routine bowel prep will ease rectal mobilization. Intraoperative insufflation of a Foley catheter within the rectum can facilitate intraoperative visualization.
    - Rectal injury is not always apparent until several days after the procedure when it may present as a retroperitoneal infection or abscess.
    - If a rectal perforation is noted intraoperatively, a general surgeon should be consulted for repair.
        - Treatment options include irrigation, direct repair, bowel rest, and antibiotics.
        - Less often, a diverting ileostomy or colostomy is necessary.
- Sacral fracture (2.9%)
    - Osteoporotic patients are at greater risk for sacral fracture.
    - A sacral fracture may present with radicular pain and may be addressed with long iliac screws.
        - If managed conservatively, there is a risk of deformity progression and worsening symptoms.
- Pelvic hematomas (2.9%)
    - Pelvic hematomas can be overlooked because of the minimally invasive nature of this approach.
        - Patients should be observed for at least 24 hours to monitor laboratory values and vital signs.
    - The presacral venous plexus, which lies just posterior to the presacral fascia, is at risk for injury during a presacral approach.
    - Typically, the bleeding is retroperitoneal and will spontaneously cease as it tamponades. The resulting hematoma will resorb.
    - If the patient becomes hemodynamically unstable, blood transfusion and vascular imaging studies should be initiated.

- Transient nerve irritation
  - Transient nerve irritation occurs infrequently and can be managed conservatively.
  - Nerve root inflammation can be avoided by strict adherence to the midline during the rod insertion.

CONCLUSION

- Axial LIF provides good clinical results, high fusion rates (90–100%), minimal blood loss, and a shorter recovery time.[1, 2]
- Axial LIF is associated with similar overall complication rates (26.5%) when compared with other fusion techniques (28–30%). However, most of the complications reported with Axial LIF (rectal perforation, sacral fracture, and pelvic hematoma) are specific to a presacral approach and may have severe consequences.[3]
- The Axial LIF provides a stable construct and high fusion rates at the lumbosacral junction in long constructs for deformity correction.[4]
- The more novel two-level Axial LIF has demonstrated to be a safe and effective surgical procedure with good short-term clinical results. However, radiolucency at the L4–L5 and L5–S1 segments, suggesting nonunion, have been reported in as many as 78.6% of patients.[5] Thus, further long-term outcomes studies are warranted to determine the efficacy and safety of this two-level axial construct.

REFERENCES

1. Gerzten PC, Tobler W, Raley TJ, Miller LE, Block JE, Nasca RJ. Axial presacral lumbar interbody fusion and percutaneous posterior fixation for stabilization of lumbosacral isthmic spondylolisthesis. J Spinal Disord Tech. 2012;25: E36-40.
2. Tobler WD, Gerszten PC, Bradley WD, et al. Minimally invasive axial presacral L5-S1 interbody fusion: two-year clinical and radiographic outcomes. Spine (Phila Pa 1976). 2011;36:E1296-301.
3. Lindley EM, McCullough MA, Burger EL, Brown CW, Patel VV. Complications of axial lumbar interbody fusion. J Neurosurg Spine. 2011;15:273-79.
4. Anand N, Baron EM, Khandehroo B, Kahwaty S. Long-term 2- to 5-year clinical and functional outcomes of minimally invasive surgery for adult scoliosis. Spine (Phila Pa 1976). 2013;38:1566-75.
5. Marchi L, Oliveira L, Coutinho E, Pimenta L. Results and complications after 2-level axial lumbar interbody fusion with a minimum 2-year follow-up. J Neurosurg Spine. 2012;17:187-92.

REFERENCE SUMMARY

1. Gerzten PC, Tobler W, Raley TJ, Miller LE, Block JE, Nasca RJ. Axial presacral lumbar interbody fusion and percutaneous posterior fixation for stabilization of lumbosacral isthmic spondylolisthesis. J Spinal Disord Tech. 2012;25: E36-E40.

   Summary: Twenty-six patients with L5-S1 spondylolisthesis (grade 1–2) were treated with an Axial LIF and percutanous posterior instrumentation. The authors reported minimal blood loss and a short hospital stay. At the 2-year follow-up, 81% of patients demonstrated excellent to good clinical results, and all patients demonstrated a radiographic arthrodesis.

2. Tobler WD, Gerszten PC, Bradley WD, Raley TJ, Nasca RJ, Block JE. Minimally invasive axial presacral L5-S1 interbody fusion: two-year clinical and radiographic outcomes. Spine (Phila Pa 1976). 2011;36:E1296-1301.
   Summary: Retrospective review of 156 patients who underwent an L5–S1 interbody fusion through a presacral approach. The authors reported significant improvement in back pain (86% of patients) and functional impairment (74% of patients). The patients demonstrated a 2-year fusion rate of 94%.
3. Lindley EM, McCullough MA, Burger EL, Brown CW, Patel VV. Complications of axial lumbar interbody fusion. Journal of Neurosurgery Spine. 2011;15:273-9.
   Summary: Retrospective review of complications associated with an Axial LIF. Of the 68 patients, 16 (23.5%) experienced complications including pseudarthrosis, superficial infection, sacral fracture, pelvic hematoma transient nerve root irritation, and rectal perforation. The authors concluded that although the complication rate is relatively low, the types of complications were approach specific and potentially severe.
4. Anand N, Baron EM, Khandehroo B, Kahwaty S. Long-term 2- to 5-year clinical and functional outcomes of minimally invasive surgery for adult scoliosis. Spine (Phila Pa 1976). 2013;38:1566-75.
   Summary: A retrospective review of 71 patients who underwent a staged MIS spinal deformity correction with the combination of a DLIF, Axial LIF, and posterior instrumentation. The authors reported good clinical and radiographic outcomes and low complication rates (22.9%). The authors suggest that an axial rod at the L5–S1 segment offers a solid fixation at the bottom of a long construct.
5. Marchi L, Oliveira L, Coutinho E, Pimenta L. Results and complications after 2-level axial lumbar interbody fusion with a minimum 2-year follow-up. Journal of Neurosurgery Spine. 2012;17:187-92.
   Summary: A prospective, nonrandomized study of 27 patients who underwent an L4–S1 Axial LIF. The authors reported intraoperative complications and one medical postoperative complication (septicemia). Despite significant clinical improvement, imaging studies demonstrated instrument-related complications including rod detachment, radiolucency around the rod, and cephalic migration. At the 2-year follow-up, only 22% of the treated levels demonstrated radiographic arthrodesis.

Chapter

13 Minimally Invasive Spine Deformity Correction

Kern Singh, Neel Anand, Alejandro Marquez-Lara, Safdar N Khan

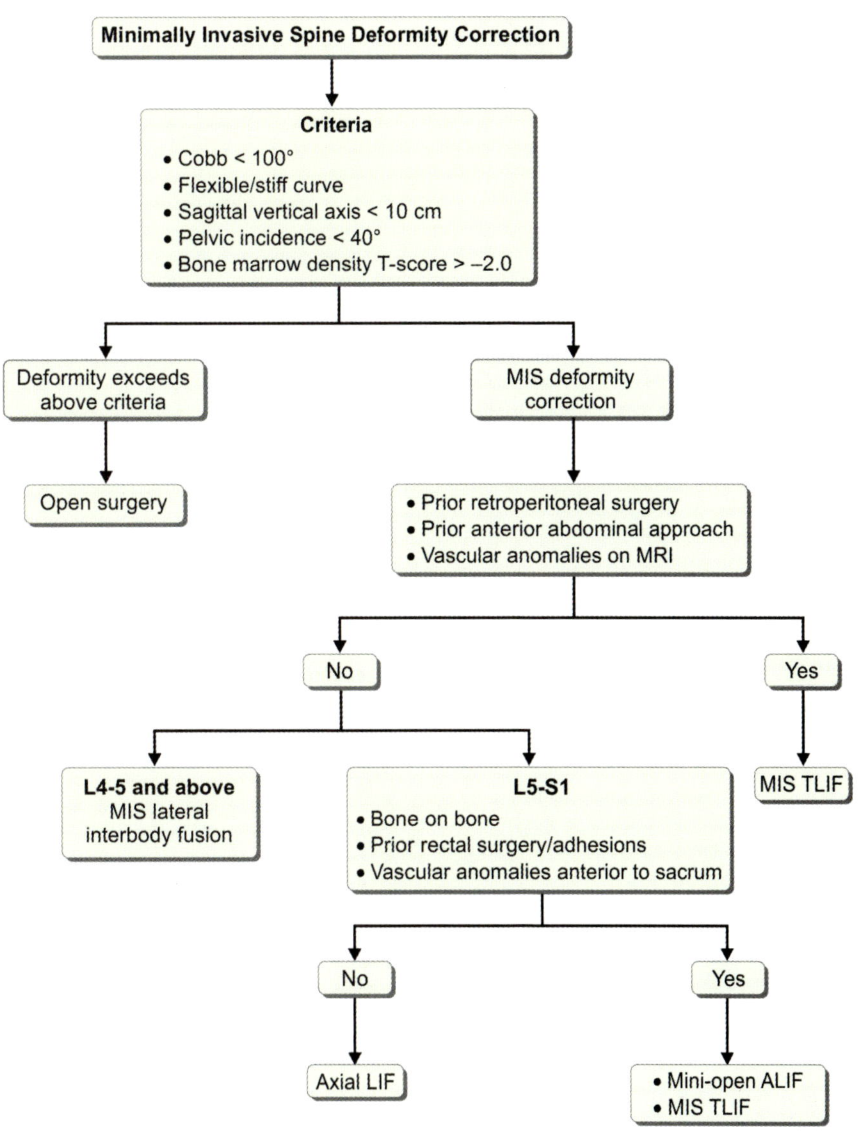

CASE VIGNETTE

A 72-year-old woman is brought to the office by her daughter for lower back pain, leg pain, and stiffness. The patient states that the pain increases with activity and worsens toward the end of the day. In addition, the patient states that after standing or walking for a prolonged period, she experiences pain and weakness in her legs requiring her to sit down. Imaging studies demonstrate a lumbar curve of 25° with an associated L5–S1 grade I spondylolisthesis on the standing radiographs and spinal stenosis on magnetic resonance imaging (MRI).

PRINCIPLES OF MINIMALLY INVASIVE DEFORMITY CORRECTION

- The goals of adult deformity correction surgery include obtaining sagittal/coronal balance and achieving a solid, stable fusion to prevent curve progression.
- Traditional open anterior, posterior, or combined approaches for adult thoracolumbar degenerative deformity are effective in correcting the sagittal and coronal alignment but are associated with significant morbidity.
  - Anterior lumbar interbody fusion (ALIF) is associated with potential risk for injury to the ureters, vasculature, bowel and parasympathetic plexus (retrograde ejaculation).
  - Posterior lumbar interbody fusion (PLIF) is associated with greater blood loss, muscle denervation, neural injury, and postoperative pain as well as proximal junctional kyphosis (PJK).
- Minimally invasive techniques provide effective deformity correction with reduced blood loss, postoperative complication rates as well as the theoretic advantage of reducing PJK.

DIAGNOSTIC IMAGING

Plain Film Radiography

- An anteroposterior (AP) and lateral full-length 36-inch standing film is obtained on all patients to analyze sagittal and coronal alignment (Figs. 13.1A and B).
  - Coronal balance: On an AP radiograph, a plumb line is dropped from the middle of the C7 vertebral body. If the line passes >1 cm from the middle of the S1 body coronal imbalance is present.
  - Sagittal balance: On a lateral radiograph, a plumb line is dropped from the middle of C7. If the line passes >–5 cm (anterior or posterior) from the posterior-superior corner of S1 sagittal imbalance is present.
  - Thoracic kyphosis: On a lateral radiograph, a Cobb angle is measured utilizing the cephalad endplate of T2 and the caudad endplate of T12. Normal range is 10°–40° (Fig. 13.2A).
  - Lumbar lordosis: On a lateral radiograph, a Cobb angle is measured utilizing the cephalad endplate of T12 and endplate of S1. Normal range is 40°–60° (Fig. 13.2B).

Imaging Pearls

- AP spine radiograph should include the C7 vertebra, sacrum, and iliac crests.
- Intraoperative fluoroscopy combined with stealth navigation can help reduce the amount of radiation exposure for surgeons and patients.

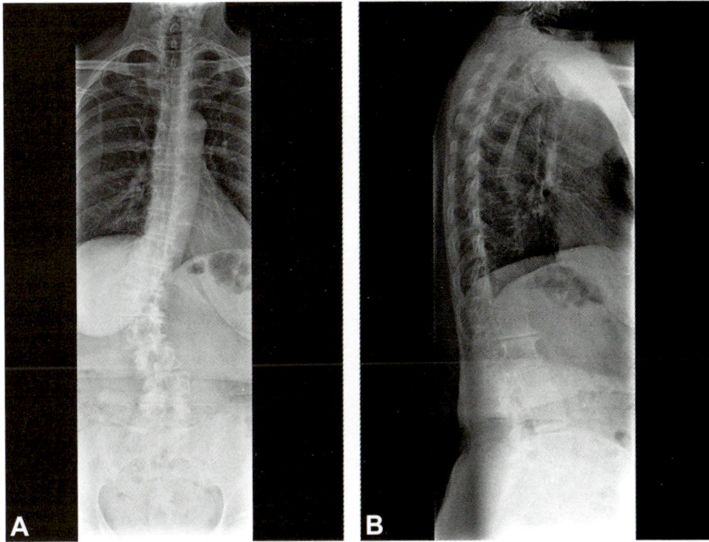

Figs. 13.1A and B: Preoperative (A) anteroposterior and (B) lateral 36-inch standing films demonstrating degenerative scoliosis.

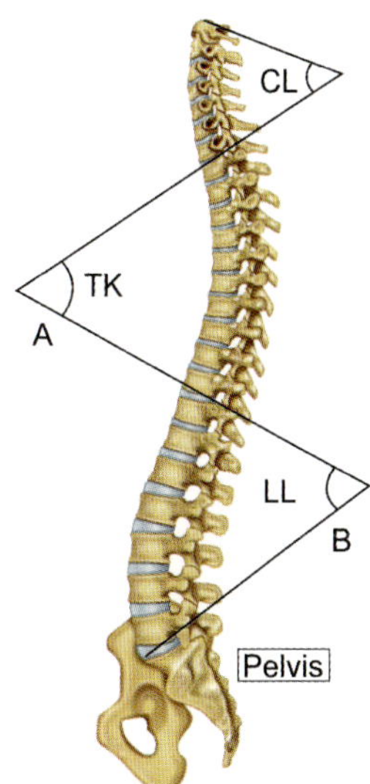

Figs. 13.2A and B: Diagram demonstrating the lines that measure the (A) thoracic kyphosis (TK) and (B) lumbar lordosis (LL).[1]

- Pelvic parameters
  - Pelvic incidence (PI): The angle that results from a line perpendicular to the sacral endplate at its midpoint and a line connecting that endplate midpoint to the femoral rotational axis (PI = PT + SS) (Fig. 13.3A).
  - Pelvic tilt (PT): The angle between the line connecting the midpoint of the sacral endplate to the femoral rotational axis and the line extending vertically from the femoral rotational axis (Fig. 13.3B).
  - Sacral slope (SS): The angle between the endplate of S1 and a horizontal line extending from the anterior-inferior corner of the S1 endplate (Fig. 13.3C).
- AP bending films assess the flexibility of the spine. If the curve corrects to <25°, the curve is considered nonstructural in nature and by definition is not included in the fusion.
- Underlying vertebral anomalies can also be assessed during the initial radiographic evaluation.
- Flexion and extension films can help analyze the amount of passive correction and dynamic instability. This information is helpful in determining the extent of the fusion necessary especially if the deformity is accompanied by listhesis.

MAGNETIC RESONANCE IMAGING

- Provides assessment of the intervertebral discs and neural compression
- MRI can detect aberrant vascular anatomy (Fig. 13.4).
- Precise coronal cuts from an MRI can demonstrate the transition between the affected and normal level, thus determining the extent of decompression and fusion.

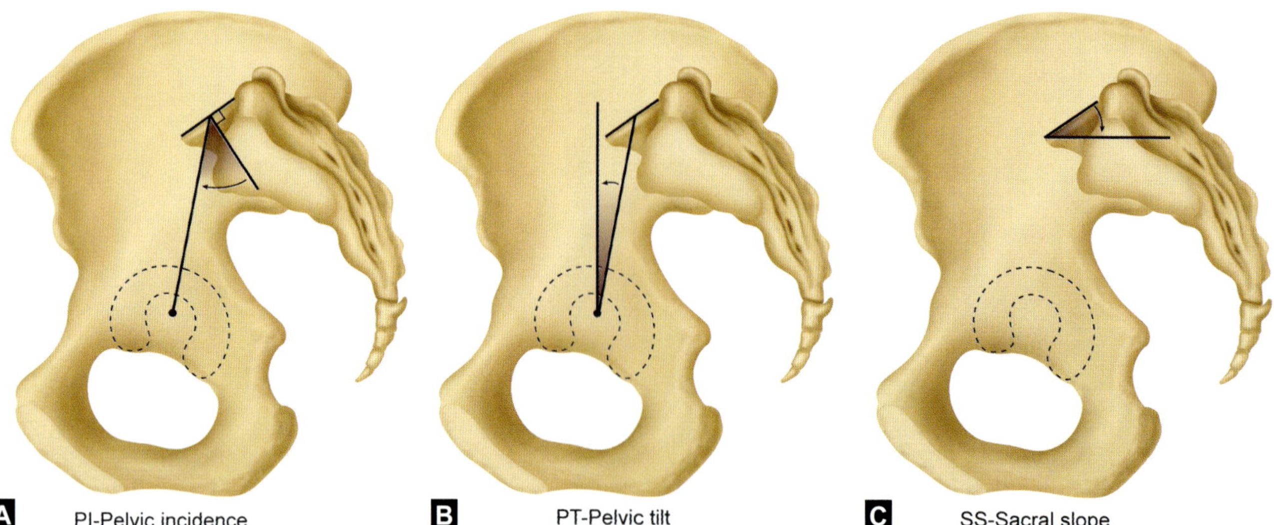

Figs. 13.3A to C: Diagrams demonstrating the lines that make up the (A) pelvic incidence, (B) pelvic tilt, and (C) sacral slope.[1] Pelvic incidence = the angle between the femoral axis and the line perpendicular to the sacral plate at the midpoint. Pelvic tilt = the angle between the line drawn from the midpoint of the sacral plate to the femoral axis and the vertical plane. Sacral slope = angle between the sacral plate and the horizontal plane.

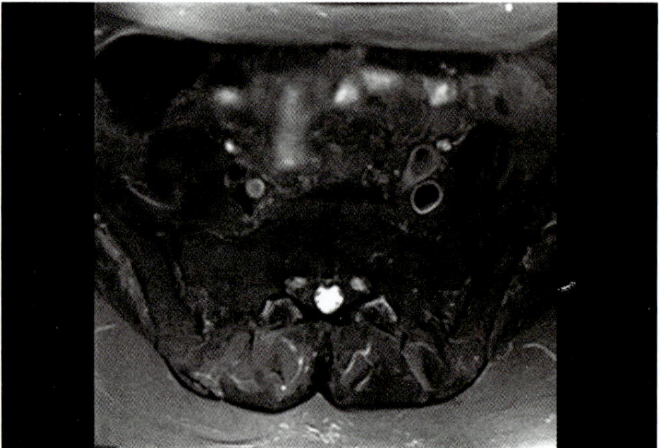

Fig. 13.4: A preoperative magnetic resonance imaging of the sacrum demonstrating the midline without aberrant vasculature.

COMPUTED TOMOGRAPHY (CT)

- A CT scan will help assess if any of the spinal segments have autofused.
- Helps determine the size and trajectory of the pedicles.
- A CT-myelography will allow precise analysis of the dural sac and neural compression.
  - CT myelography is indicated in those patients with prior spinal instrumenation and complaints of continued radicular pain.

Bone Scintigraphy

- A bone scan should be performed on patients >50 years of age. If the T-score is <–2.0, a minimally invasive approach should not be performed.

Surgical Indications

- Spinal deformity with symptomatic back and/or leg pain.
  - Scoliosis
    - Degenerative
    - Idiopathic
    - Syndromic
    - Iatrogenic
- Deformity progression
- Flexible curves
- Cobb angle 10°–60°
- Radiculopathy (foraminal stenosis on the side of the concavity of the curve)
- Lumbar hyperlordosis
- Fixed lateral listhesis with preserved motion on side bending films.
- Spinal stenosis

Indication Pearls

- Conservative therapy including bracing, epidural, and facet injections, and physical therapy should be exhausted prior to surgical intervention.

Contraindications

- Fixed sagittal imbalance > 10 cm
- High-grade spondylolisthesis (grade III or greater)
- Rigid curves
- Cobb angle > 60°
- Pelvic incidence > 40°

Surgical Decision Making

Understanding the etiology, anatomy, and clinical presentation of the spinal deformity will help guide surgical management.

- Degenerative Scoliosis
  - Etiology: Develops from a combination of spinal degenerative changes with asymmetric disc collapse, facet joint degeneration, spondylolisthesis, and subluxation.
  - Anatomy: The deformity is located in the lumbar spine and rarely involves the thoracic spine. Despite a rotary subluxation, the typical large rotational deformity is generally not present. However, lateral listhesis is more common in this patient population. Typically, L4 slides off L5 and L3 rotates off L4.
  - Clinical presentation: Patients who require surgery will demonstrate a declining quality of life from neurological symptoms including radiculopathy, claudication, and progressive, worsening back pain.
  - Surgical management: Lumbar decompression and fusion techniques are typically utilized.
- Adult idiopathic scoliosis with superimposed degenerative changes
  - Etiology: This anomaly results from degenerative changes to a pre-existing adolescent scoliosis.
  - Anatomy: These patients will typically have a more severe deformity (increased rotatory deformity) involving both the thoracic and lumbar spine.
  - Clinical presentation: These patients are in their 4th or 5th decade and present with severe lower and midback pain and complain of significant coronal and sagittal misalignment.

Pearls

- A fixed deformity will likely require a shortening procedure via an open osteotomy (i.e. Smith-Peterson, pedicle subtraction). However, percutaneous pedicle screw fixation techniques for posterior stabilization can be combined with these open procedures.

Surgical Management

- If spinal stenosis is present, anterior column decompression (indirect) is effective at relieving symptoms. Thus, an extensive laminectomy (direct decompression) with its associated posterior soft tissue trauma and extensive blood loss is avoided.

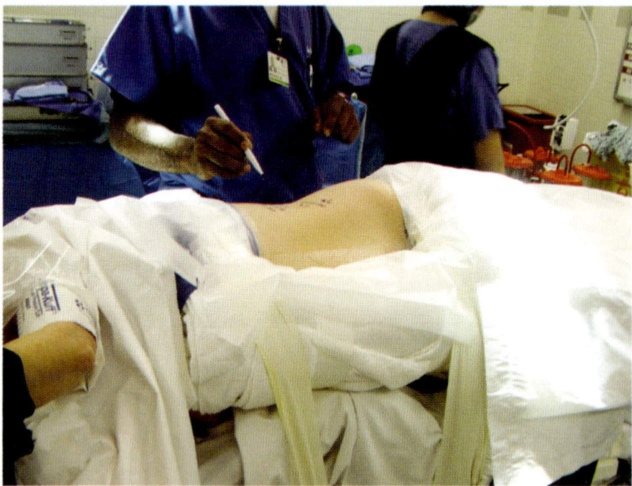

Fig. 13.5: A patient placed in a lateral decubitus position in preparation for a lateral lumbar interbody fusion. Note the bump at the target level to maximize the distance between the iliac crest and rib cage.

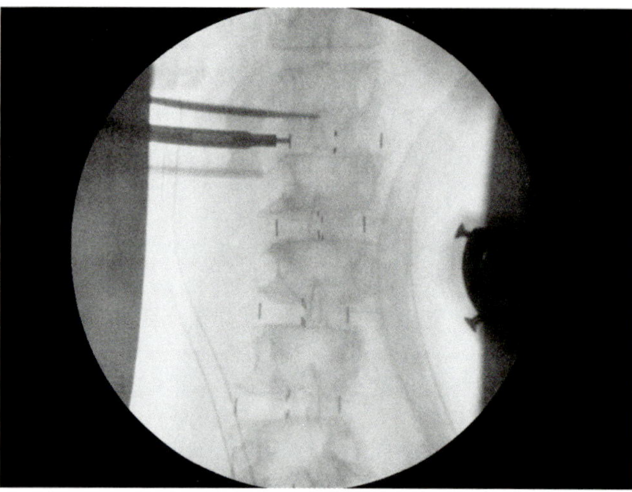

Fig. 13.6: Intraoperative anteroposterior fluoroscopic image demonstrating a PEEK cage being impacted into position. Several cages have already been placed in the lower levels.

- Anterior column reconstruction and fusion can be achieved with multiple minimally invasive techniques [Axial LIF, transforaminal LIF (TLIF), lateral LIF (LLIF), mini-ALIF] by utilizing interbody spacers and bone grafts and/or substitutes.
  - Critical to the success of these techniques is the placement of the interbody spacer along the cortical rim or apophyseal ring, which are the strongest portions of the endplate.
- Posterior percutaneous pedicle screw fixation is a safe, efficient, and effective technique for posterior stabilization. The extent of the deformity and symptoms will dictate the length of the construct.

SURGICAL TECHNIQUES

- The lateral transpsoas approach (LLIF) can be utilized to address most levels above L5–S1 (Fig. 13.5).
  - Up to three levels can be accessed through a single incision.
  - An interbody spacer that provides initial stability and a solid scaffold for bony in growth should be utilized (Fig. 13.6) (i.e. PEEK or tantalum cages).
  - Several bone graft options are available as an adjunct for arthrodesis. Bone autograft (harvested or local), demineralized bone matrix, and other graft substitutes (rhBMP-2) are effective at achieving a solid fusion.
  - For prolonged cases involving multiple levels, staging the posterior pedicle screw fixation to 2–3 days after the index LLIF can help evaluate patients for signs of adequate neurological decompression.
    - A repeat 36-inch plain film radiograph should also be obtained in between stages to reassess the coronal and sagittal parameters so as to plan for the necessary correction.

Pearls

- The LLIF approach enables placement of larger interbody spacers, thereby providing a greater degree of deformity correction when compared with other MIS techniques (TLIF, ALIF).
- If pelvic fixation is required, bilateral S2 alar-iliac (S2AI) screws can be placed utilizing a teardrop view.
- All levels within the Cobb angle are instrumented. If the fusion crosses the thoracolumbar junction, it is stopped at the first normal parallel disc irrespective of whether it is at L1–T12 or T11.

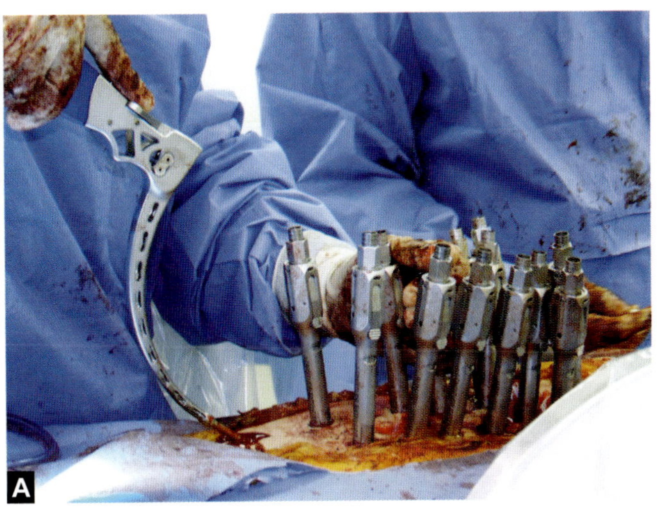

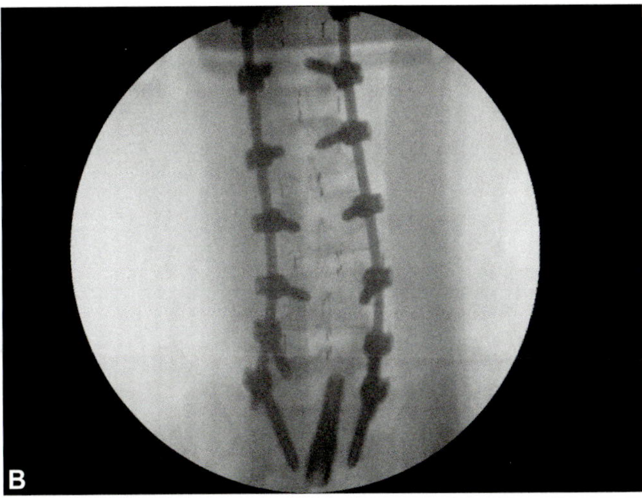

Figs. 13.7A and B: (A) A rod is being passed on a rod holder percutaneously through pedicle screw extenders. (B) Anteroposteior radiograph demonstrating a final construct with percutaneously inserted pedicle screws and rods, one level distracting axial rod, and several interbody cages.

- An L5–S1 level fusion can be achieved through several approaches. The decision will depend upon the surgeon's preference, technique limitations, and the potential contraindications.
  - Presacral (Axial LIF)
    - This is a technically challenging procedure with a limited potential for reduction and distraction. Potential for rectal injury.
    - Contraindicated in patients with previous pelvic surgery, presacral scarring, and presacral vascular anomalies.
  - Anterior (mini-open)
    - This approach enables adequate decompression and fusion at the L5–S1 level but requires changing the patient's position if a posterior decompression and/or instrumentation is required.
    - This approach is contraindicated in patients with previous abdominal surgeries or aberrant abdominal vasculature.
  - Posterior (TLIF)
    - Minimally invasive surgical (MIS) TLIF achieves anterior column decompression and fusion while providing access to the posterior elements without changing the patient's position.
    - This technically challenging procedure has a steep learning curve. In addition, it may not be as effective in cases with an associated high-grade spondylolisthesis.
- Posterior percutaneous pedicle screw fixation (unilateral or bilateral) is often utilized for additional stability (Figs. 13.7A and B).
  - Pedicle screw fixation and rod placement is critical in achieving the desired curvature correction.
    - Individual paramedian skin and fascial incisions are made for each pedicle screw that is placed.
    - Alternatively, a single longitudinal midline skin incision with individual paramedian fascial incisions can also be utilized for screw placement.

Pearls

- Injecting bone cement into the pedicles prior to screw placement will increase fixation strength in patients with osteoporotic bone.

Pitfalls

- Screw malalignment can lead to screw pull during the reduction maneuver. This is particularly prevalent at the lumbosacral junction.

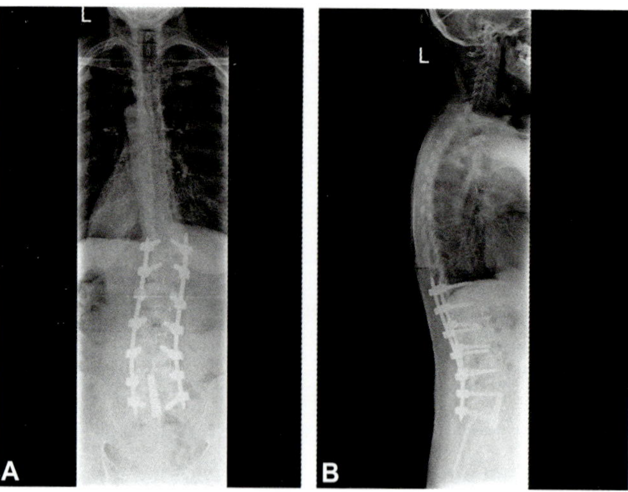

Figs. 13.8A and B: Postoperative 36-inch standing films demonstrating good coronal and sagittal balance and good deformity correction.

- If an LLIF approach is undertaken, unilateral pedicle screws can be placed in the lateral decubitus position.
- Alternatively, patients can be repositioned into a prone position to place bilateral pedicle screws, which provide a greater correction of the curvature.
- After screw placement, a rod of the appropriate size and contour is passed percutaneously through the screw heads. Curve reduction can then be performed in a caudal to rostral direction with care to maintain the rod in a strict sagittal orientation.
  - Facet joint release during the index decompression and fusion procedure will facilitate curve reduction.

CONCLUSION

- Understanding the surgical indications for addressing adult spinal deformity will enable appropriate patient selection and better outcomes.
- An LLIF for the management of adult degenerative scoliosis is associated with a significant improvement in disease specific and quality-of-life outcome measures. In addition, minimally invasive deformity correction is associated with a reduced procedural time, less blood loss, shorter hospital stay, and reduced complication rates when compared with open techniques.[1-3]
- Radiographic deformity correction and high fusion rates (98%) can be achieved via a minimally invasive surgical approach (LLIF). However, supplemental posterior fixation is often necessary to provide the greatest coronal and sagittal correction[1] (Figs. 13.8A and B).

REFERENCES

1. Phillips FM, Isaacs RE, Rodgers WB, et al. Adult degenerative scoliosis treated with XLIF: clinical and radiographic results of a prospective multi-center study with 24-month follow-up. Spine (Phila Pa 1976). 2013;38(21):1853-61.
2. Isaacs RE HJ, Goodrich JA, Rodgers WB, Phillips FM. A prospective, non-randomized, multicenter evaluation of extreme lateral interbody fusion for the treatment of adult degenerative scoliosis—perioperative outcomes and complications. Spine. 2010;35:S322-30.
3. Dakwar E, Cardona RF, Smith DA, Uribe JS. Early outcomes and safety of the minimally invasive, lateral retroperitoneal transpsoas approach for adult degenerative scoliosis. Neurosurg Focus. 2010;28:E8.

REFERENCE SUMMARY

1. Phillips FM, Isaacs RE, Rodgers WB, et al. Adult degenerative scoliosis treated with XLIF: clinical and radiographic results of a prospective multi-center study with 24-month follow-up. Spine (Phila Pa 1976). 2013;38(21):1853-61.
   Summary: A prospective nonrandomized muticenter study ($n = 107$) evaluating the clinical and radiographic outcomes of an LLIF for the treatment of adult scoliosis. The authors reported a sustained improvement in the clinical outcomes measures with a persistent sagittal and coronal deformity correction and fusion. The LLIF is associated with fewer complications than traditional open procedures with similar clinical and radiographic outcomes.
2. Isaacs RE HJ, Goodrich JA, Rodgers WB, Phillips FM. A prospective, non-randomized, multicenter evaluation of extreme lateral interbody fusion for the treatment of adult degenerative scoliosis—perioperative outcomes and complications. Spine. 2010;35:S322-S330.
   Summary: A prospective nonrandomized multicenter study ($n = 107$) evaluating the clinical and radiographic outcomes of an LLIF for the treatment of degenerative scoliosis. The authors reported an avergae operative time of 178 minutes, blood loss of 50–100cm^3, and a postoperative complication rate of 12.1%. The authors concluded that the LLIF technique reduces the morbidity associated with traditional open spinal deformity correction procedures.
3. Dakwar E, Cardona RF, Smith DA, Uribe JS. Early outcomes and safety of the minimally invasive, lateral retroperitoneal transpsoas approach for adult degenerative scoliosis. Neurosurgical Focus 2010;28:E8.
   Summary: A retrospective review of 25 patients who underwent anterior column reconstruction for degenerative scoliosis through a lateral transpsoas approach. The authors reported an average blood loss of 53 cm^3 and a hospital stay of 6.2 days. Postoperative complications (24%) included transient anterior thigh numbness, rhabdomyolysis, graft subsidence, and hardware failure. The authors conlcuded that a minimally invasive lateral transpsoas approach is a feasible alternative for the restoration of disc height, arthrodesis, and realignment for degenerative scoliosis.

Chapter

14

Minimally Invasive Spinal Tumor Resection

Kern Singh, Sreeharsha V Nandyala, Hamid Hassanzadeh, Alexander R Vaccaro

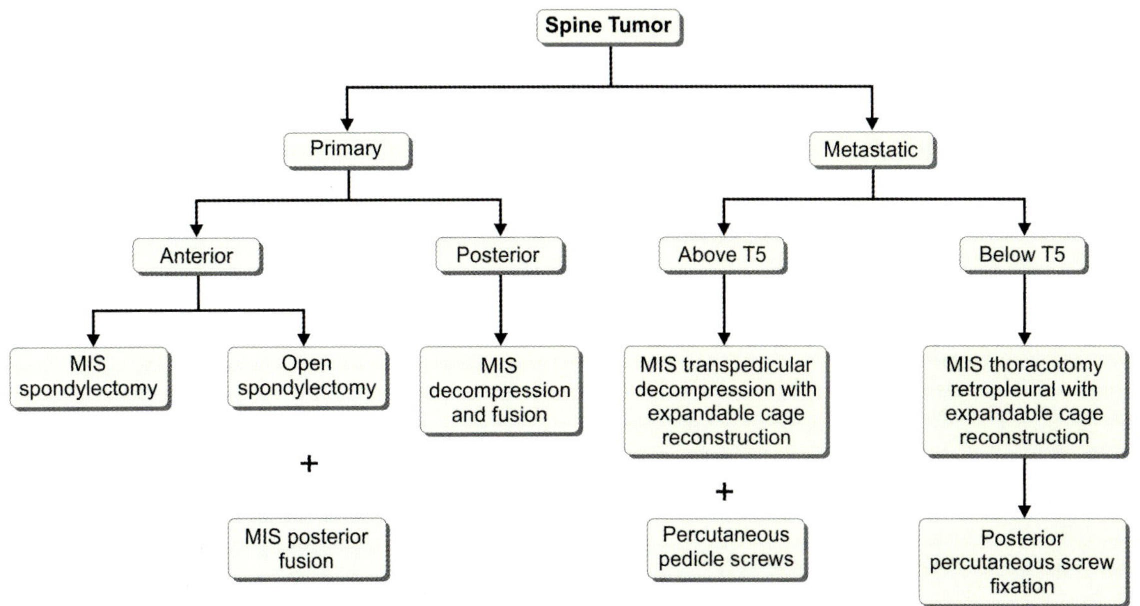

CASE VIGNETTE

A 35-year-old woman with a history of breast cancer presents to the office with worsening mid back pain. The patient states that the pain is constant, worsens at night, and is not associated with activity. She denies any numbness, weakness, or bowel or bladder incontinence. Medical management has provided minimal relief. On physical examination, the patient demonstrates a correctable kyphotic posture but no motor or sensory deficit.

PRINCIPLES OF MINIMALLY INVASIVE SPINAL TUMOR RESECTION

- Spinal tumors (primary or metastatic) may be associated with significant pain and axial spine instability thereby limiting mobility.
- The goals of spinal oncologic surgery are to achieve complete tumor resection, relieve pain, and preserve or restore spinal stability and neurologic function.[1,2]

Pearls

- Two thirds of spine metastases are from advanced breast and prostate cancer.
- Prolonged postoperative immobilization after an extensive surgical intervention increases the risk for a thromboembolic event in patients who are already in a hypercoagulable state. Thromboprophylaxis should be utilized in this very high-risk patient population.

- It is essential for the surgical approach to provide access to the anterior column for decompression and stabilization since 70% of spinal metastases involve the vertebral body.
- Traditional spinal tumor resection is associated with a large and extensive surgical dissection, significant blood loss, infection risk, and postoperative debilitation.

DIAGNOSTIC IMAGING

- Magnetic resonance imaging (MRI)
  - An MRI is the most sensitive and specific test for the diagnosis of a spinal tumor.
  - It is recommended to obtain an MRI of the entire axial spine to detect multiple lesions and to help guide potential radiotherapy (RT) planning.
    - For patients who cannot undergo an MRI study (cardiac pacemakers or ocular implants) a computed tomography (CT)-myelography is an acceptable alternative.
- Computed tomography
  - A CT can demonstrate areas of vertebral destruction and help assess the adjacent osseous anatomy for surgical planning.
  - This imaging modality has a relatively low sensitivity (66%), for which its utilization for diagnosis is limited.
- Bone scintigraphy
  - A bone scan is a sensitive test that can detect tumors as small as 2 mm in size and 3–18 months earlier than a plain film radiograph.
  - However, it has a low sensitivity for osteolytic lesions (multiple myeloma, renal cell carcinoma) and does not provide an accurate anatomic level.
- Positron emission tomography (PET)/CT
  - PET/CT can be utilized for the initial staging of the tumor. It has a higher sensitivity, specificity, and a negative predictive value than a bone scintigraphy.
- Plain film radiography
  - Plain film radiography will detect changes in the trabecular bone after 30–50% of bony destruction. Therefore, the utilization of this study for diagnosis is not indicated.
  - Plain film radiography allows for the assessment of spinal alignment and stability as well as for the evaluation of pathologic fractures.
  - Serial radiographs can also be utilized to monitor the disease progression in patients who are conservatively managed.

SURGICAL INDICATIONS

- Curative—For benign or malignant primary tumors without perivertebral soft tissue invasion
- Palliative—For malignant primary tumors with perivertebral soft tissue invasion or metastatic disease
  - Intractable pain
  - Spinal instability

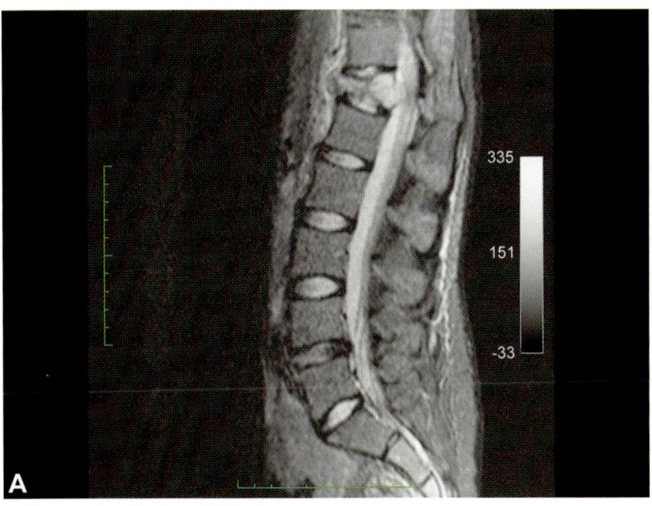

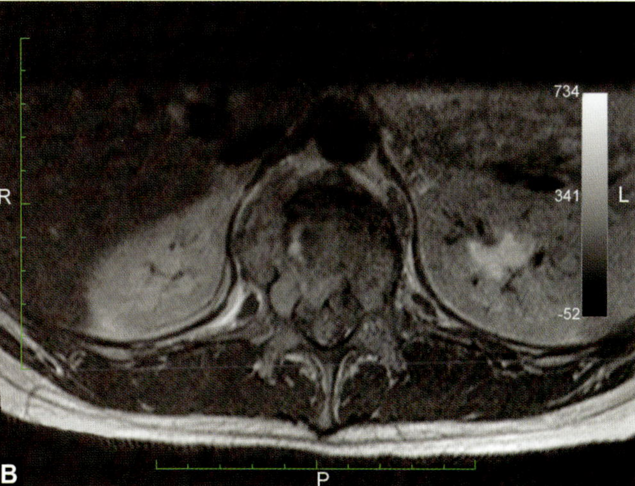

Figs. 14.1A and B: (A) Preoperative sagittal magnetic resonance imaging (MRI) demonstrating a locally destructive tumor in the L1 vertebral body causing collapse with local kyphosis. (B) Axial MRI of the same patient where the tumor is visualized compressing the neural elements.

- Progressive neurological deficit
- Radioresistant tumors (i.e. renal cell carcinoma and melanoma)

SURGICAL DECISION MAKING

The appropriate surgical intervention is based upon the tumor biology and stage, spinal stability, neurological status, and the disease burden.

- Tumor biology and stage
  - Primary benign tumors (osteoblastoma, hemangioma, eosinophilic granuloma)
    - Rarely require surgical management
    - When surgery is indicated, wide margins are not required with surgical resection.
  - Primary malignant tumors (osteosarcoma, Ewing's sarcoma, chondrosarcoma)
    - En bloc resection with wide surgical margins is indicated when there is no evidence of perivertebral soft tissue invasion or distant metastases.
    - Adjuvant RT and chemotherapy is often utilized.
  - Metastases
    - Curative—Spondylectomy or corpectomy
    - Palliative—Transpedicular decompression or cement augmentation
    - Local vasculature involvement will affect the feasibility of the tumor resection.
- Spinal stability
  - The extent of bone loss is a critical factor that affects the stability of the spine.
    - Vertebral body collapse, segmental deformity, and posterior element involvement are indications for spinal arthrodesis (Figs. 14.1A and B).

Pearls

- Highly vascularized tumors (renal cell carcinoma, papillary thyroid carcinoma, and melanoma) may benefit from a preoperative angiography and selective tumor embolization to reduce intraoperative blood loss.

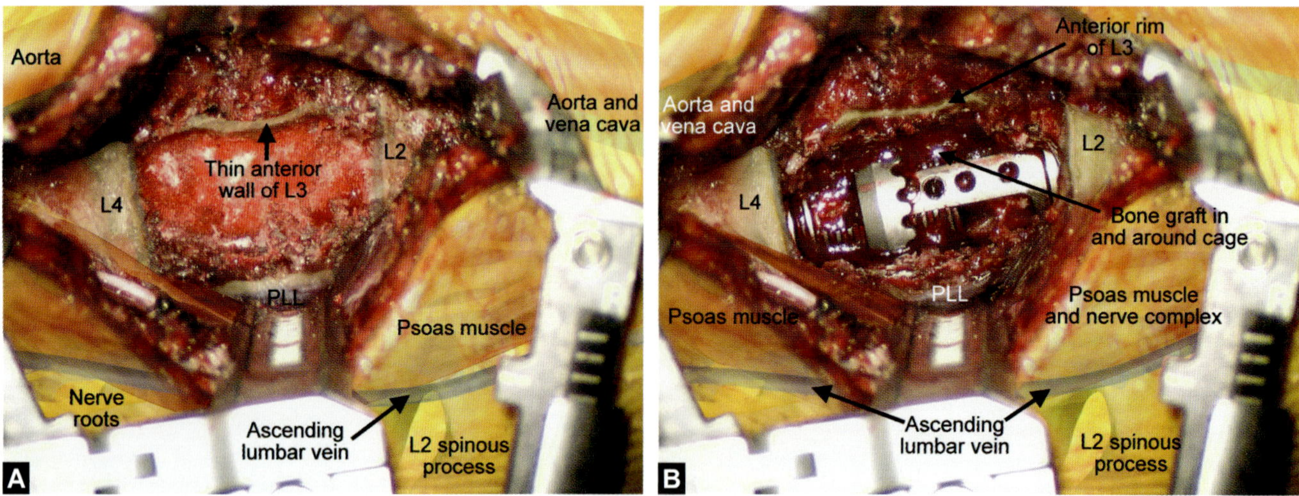

Figs. 14.2A and B: (A) Intraoperative view of a minimally invasive lateral approach for a lumbar corpectomy. (B) The defect is reconstructed with an expandable titanium cage.

- Neurological status
  - Patients with acute to subacute neurological deficit will benefit from complete decompression of the spinal cord. Thus, the location of the spinal cord compression will determine the surgical approach.
- Disease burden
  - Although difficult to predict, a patient's disease burden and the expected survival period allows the assessment of the overall risks associated with a surgical intervention.
  - Patients with a significant disease burden may benefit from non-surgical management and palliative care.

THE SURGICAL APPROACH

- Primary spinal tumors without neurological deficit
  - The location of the tumor will determine the surgical approach.
  - The severity of instability after the tumor resection will determine the need for an instrumented stabilization.
    - This can be achieved through a percutaneous pedicle screw fixation.
  - En bloc resection is an appropriate surgical option for malignant tumors that are completely contained within the vertebral body (Figs. 14.2A and B).
    - A traditional open surgical approach is often indicated to assure a wide resection with negative margins and reduce the risk of tumor recurrence.
- Primary spinal tumors with neurological deficit
  - These tumors are generally malignant for which a formal open decompression and stabilization is required.
  - Posterior instrumentation for stabilization can also be accomplished through percutaneous pedicle screw fixation.
- Metastatic spinal tumors without neurological deficit
  - Surgical intervention is indicated in cases of spinal instability

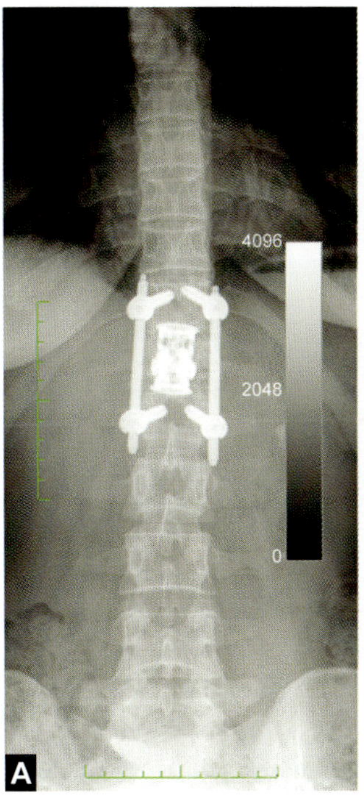

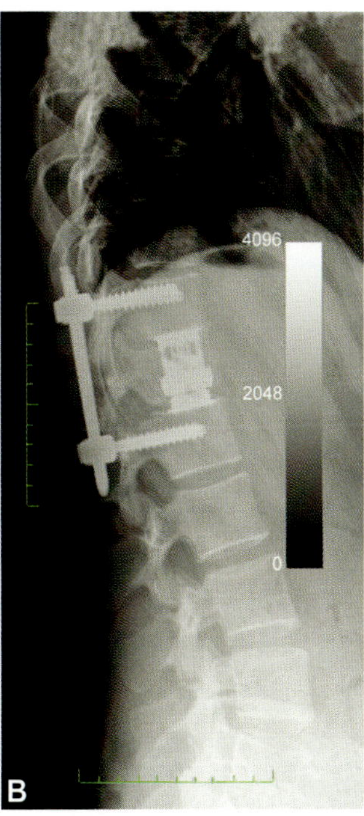

Figs. 14.3A and B: Postoperative (A) anteroposterior and (B) lateral radiographs of an L1 vertebral body reconstruction with an expandable cage after corpectomy. Posterior stabilization was achieved via percutaneous pedicle screw fixation.

- A minimally invasive anterior column reconstruction through a posterior transpedicular decompression or a retropleural/retroperitoneal approach can be performed since intralesional margins are acceptable (Figs. 14.3A and B).
- A complementary posterior fusion through percutaneous pedicle screws is utilized to provide stabilization.

- Metastatic spinal tumors with neurological deficit
  - Neurological deficit is the most common indication for surgery in patients with spinal metastases.
  - Surgical decompression should be performed (minimally invasive surgical vs open) (Fig. 14.4).
    - Above T5—A posterior transpedicular approach is preferred.
    - Below T5—A minimally invasive retropleural/retroperitoneal corpectomy can be utilized for neural decompression.
  - A posterior stabilization can be achieved with posterior percutaneous pedicle screws.

Pearls

- Radiation therapy (RT) should be delayed up to 2–3 weeks after surgery to allow for soft tissue healing. If a bone graft is utilized, RT should be delayed for up to 4–6 weeks after surgery.

THE ROLE OF VERTEBRAL BODY CEMENT AUGMENTATION—KYPHOPLASTY AND VERTEBROPLASTY

- The injection of polymethylmethacrylate (PMMA) is effective in relieving pain from spine metastases and can provide stability and strengthen the compromised vertebrae.

Pitfalls

- Contraindications to bone cement augmentation include patients with ≥75% loss of vertebral body height, ≥20% spinal canal compromise, posterior vertebral body cortex violation, more than three levels requiring treatment, radiculopathy, and/or uncorrectable coagulopathy.

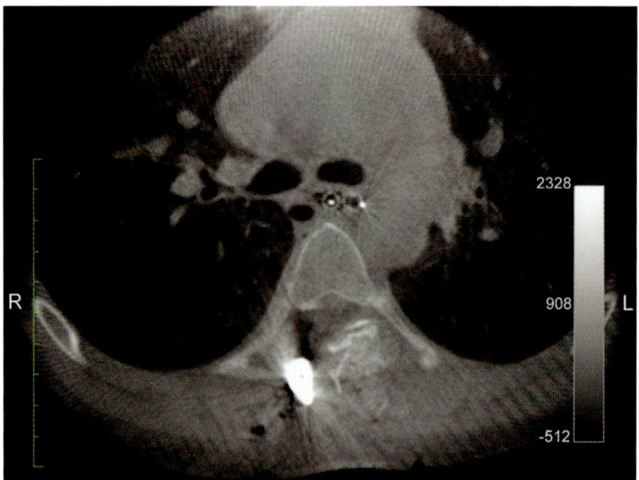

Fig. 14.4: Intraoperative O-arm imaging with navigation, which is utilized to assure adequate decompression of the spinal canal via a minimally invasive transpedicular approach.

    - A percutaneous transpedicular technique can be utilized to inject cement into the vertebral body.
    - Kyphoplasty provides the additional benefit of restoring vertebral height and correcting kyphotic deformities.
- PMMA is stable to the effects of RT so it can be performed before or after RT.

CONCLUSION

- Patients with acute to subacute neurological deficits demonstrate significant improvement in neurological function and survival with surgical treatment.[2]
- A minimally invasive approach for tumor decompression allows early postoperative initiation of adjuvant radiation therapy due to a reduced risk for wound dehiscence.[3]

REFERENCES

1. Bhatt AD, Schuler JC, Boakye M, Woo SY. Current and emerging concepts in non-invasive and minimally invasive management of spine metastasis. Cancer Treat Rev. 2013;39:142-52.
2. Patchell RA, Tibbs PA, Regine WF, et al. Direct decompressive surgical resection in the treatment of spinal cord compression caused by metastatic cancer: a randomised trial. Lancet. 2005;366:643-8.
3. Zairi F, Arikat A, Allaoui M, Marinho P, Assaker R. Minimally invasive decompression and stabilization for the management of thoracolumbar spine metastasis. J Neurosurg Spine. 2012;17:19-23.

REFERENCE SUMMARY

1. Bhatt AD, Schuler JC, Boakye M, Woo SY. Current and emerging concepts in non-invasive and minimally invasive management of spine metastasis. Cancer Treatment Reviews. 2013;39:142-52.

Summary: A literature review on the presentation, work-up, and the management of spine metastasis with or without spinal cord compression. The authors explain that the surgical management should aim to improve the patient's quality of life by preventing neurologic decline, providing durable pain relief, and local tumor control.

2. Patchell RA, Tibbs PA, Regine WF, et al. Direct decompressive surgical resection in the treatment of spinal cord compression caused by metastatic cancer: a randomised trial. The Lancet. 2005;366:643-8.

   Summary: A randomised, multicenter, nonblinded trial that compared surgery followed by radiotherapy to radiotherapy (RT) alone for the management of spinal cord compression caused by metastatic cancer. The authors demonstrated a significantly greater neurological improvement in the surgical cohort when compared with RT alone.

3. Zairi F, Arikat A, Allaoui M, Marinho P, Assaker R. Minimally invasive decompression and stabilization for the management of thoracolumbar spine metastasis. Journal of Neurosurgery Spine. 2012;17:19-23.

   Summary: A prospective case series of 10 patients with thoracolumbar metastasis who underwent a minimally invasive posterior transpedicular vertebrectomy and spinal cord decompression. The authors concluded that this minimally invasive approach is a safe and effective intervention for the palliative treatment of patients with a limited life expectancy.

Chapter

15

Minimally Invasive Surgery for Spinal Trauma

Alpesh A Patel, Alejandro Marquez-Lara, Hamid Hassanzadeh, Kern Singh

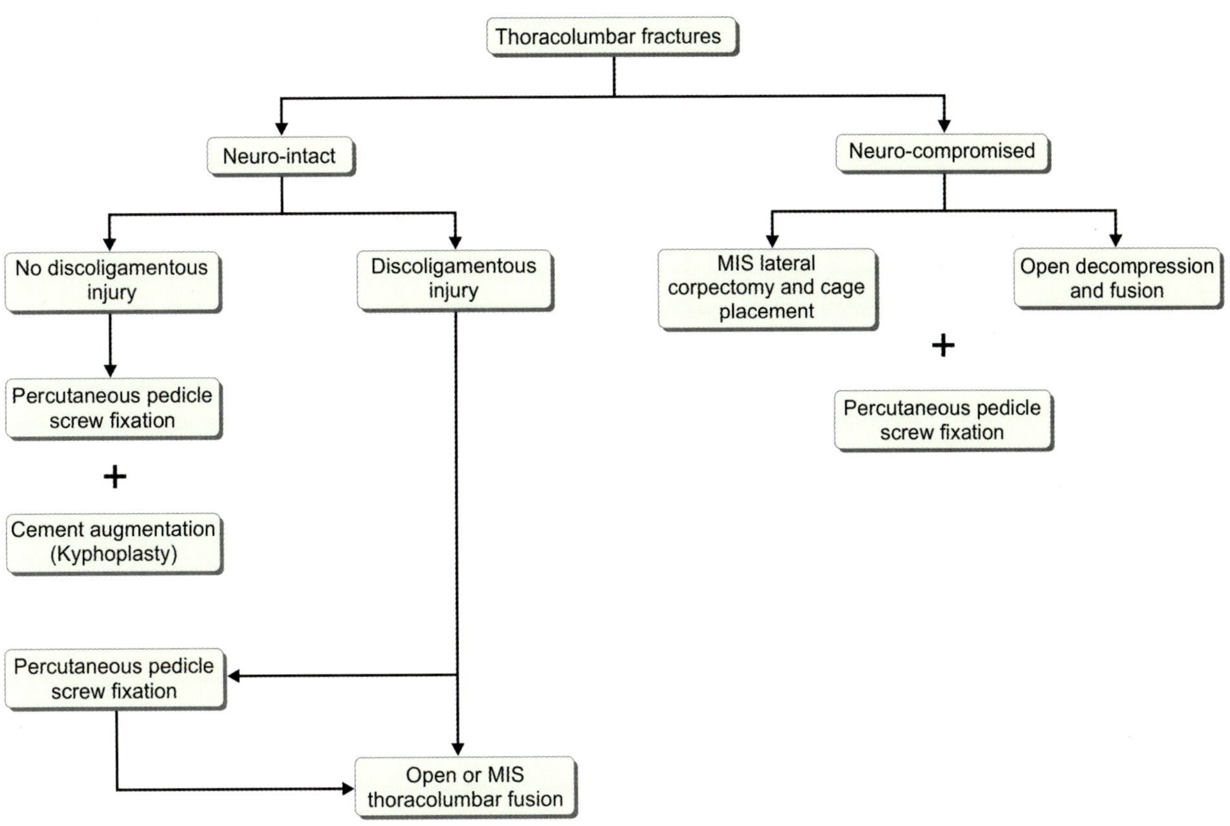

CASE VIGNETTE

A 31-year-old man presents to the emergency department after a motor vehicle accident. In the trauma bay, the patient is spontaneously moving all extremities. The patient's vital signs are stable. However, the primary survey demonstrates diminished mechanical breath sounds on the left hemithorax, palpable pulses in all extremities, and an obvious deformity on the right thigh. Rectal tone is intact. Imaging studies demonstrate a mid-femur shaft fracture, a left pneumothorax, and a flexion-distraction injury with bony and ligamentous involvement at T12-L1. After medical stabilization and treatment of the pneumothorax, the patient underwent a posterior percutaneous pedicle screw instrumentation and stabilization.

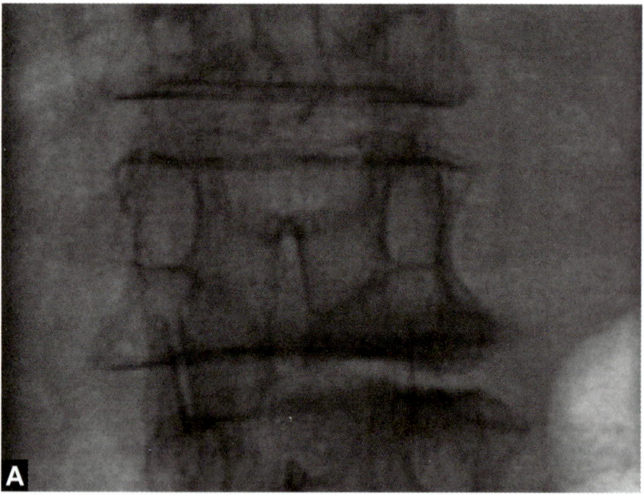

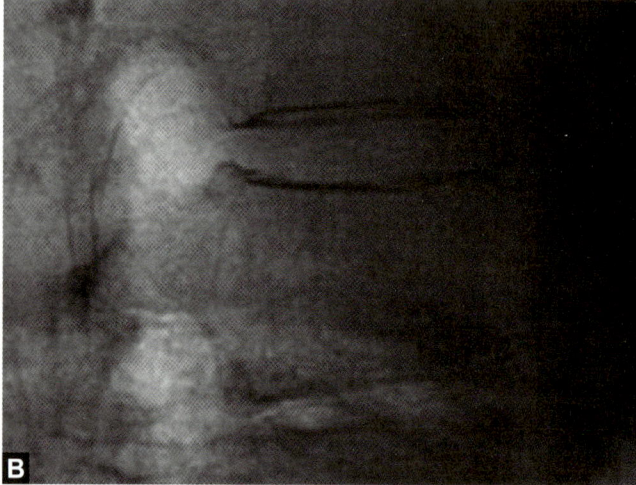

Figs. 15.1A and B: (A) A true anteroposterior radiograph of the vertebral body. The endplates are parallel and the pedicles are equidistant to the spinous process. (B) A true lateral radiograph of the vertebral body. Note the pedicles are superimposed and the superior and inferior endplates are parallel.

PRINCIPLES OF MINIMALLY INVASIVE SURGERY FOR SPINAL TRAUMA

- Surgical goals for thoracolumbar spine fractures include the restoration of spinal stability and decompression of affected neural structures to promote early mobilization and to prevent the development of post-traumatic kyphosis.
- Patients with concomitant injuries to multiple organ systems may not tolerate a prolonged open procedure due to the associated soft tissue damage, increased blood loss (>1000 cm^3), and a greater potential for infection (10%).[1]
- An open posterior approach to the thoracolumbar spine can result in muscle denervation and ischemia. This may result in significant pain and muscle weakness, which can negatively impact early postoperative rehabilitation.
- For certain injury patterns, the surgical goals for a thoracolumbar injury can be achieved through a minimally invasive approach while reducing the morbidity associated with traditional open interventions.[2,3]

Pearls

- Pedicle screws can provide immediate stability for trauma patients.
- MIS techniques may be utilized to provide provisional stability and fixation until the patient can tolerate an anterior or posterior arthrodesis.

Pitfalls

- Pedicle screw fixation is associated with increased radiation exposure.
- The benefit of a minimally invasive technique may be hindered by the steep learning curve.

DIAGNOSTIC IMAGING

- Plain film radiography (Figs. 15.1A and B)
  - Plain film radiographs provide the initial assessment of a spine fracture.
  - Plain films may not identify more subtle, nondisplaced, or minimally displaced fractures.
- Computed tomography (CT)
  - A CT scan is the most sensitive and specific test to evaluate injury morphology and inferred instability.

  - CT allows for assessment of the spinal canal and facet joint congruity.
  - The size and angulation of each pedicle can be measured to determine screw size and trajectory.
- Magnetic resonance imaging (MRI)
  - An MRI may assess the presence of ligamentous injuries as well as spinal cord and nerve root compression.

Pitfall

- MRI will have a high sensitivity but low specificity. It should not be utilized in isolation to diagnose and classify an injury.

SURGICAL INDICATIONS

- Unstable burst fractures
- Flexion-distraction injuries
- Extension-distraction injuries
- Fracture dislocations
- Unstable sacral fractures requiring lumbar-pelvic fixation

Pearls

- Early thoracolumbar stabilization (48 hours) can reduce the risk of respiratory complications in polytrauma patients.

SURGICAL DECISION MAKING

Choosing the appropriate surgical intervention is based upon the stability of the fracture (injury morphology and integrity of the posterior ligamentous complex), the patient's neurological status, and the other associated injuries:

- Spinal stability
  - Stable fracture patterns (nondisplaced burst fractures, bony chance fractures)
    - These fractures are often amenable to conservative management with external bracing.
    - In certain cases (intractable pain, obese body habitus) a posterior percutaneous pedicle screw fixation can help achieve adequate stability to allow for controlled fracture healing.
  - Unstable fracture patterns generally require reduction and fusion, which can be achieved via an open or minimally invasive approach.
    - An open reduction for complex fracture patterns can be combined with a percutaneous posterior stabilization resulting in a hybrid technique.
    - Minimally invasive surgical (MIS) techniques can be utilized to obtain provisional fixation with a staged anterior and/or posterior open arthrodesis.
- Neurological compromise
  - Fractures associated with worsening neurologic symptoms (myelopathy, cauda equina) will require a formal decompression and fusion.
    - This can be achieved via an open or minimally invasive technique depending on fracture pattern and ongoing neural compression.
    - Additional posterior stability can be provided with percutaneous pedicle screw fixation.
- Associated injuries
  - Patients who present with multiple skin abrasions near a traditional open surgical incision site can benefit from a minimally invasive fixation (Figs. 15.2A to D).

Pearls

- In the presence of ligamentous instability, the facet joints can be fused via a minimally invasive approach. Prior to the pedicle screw placement, the facet capsule is removed with an electrocautery. A high-speed burr can be used to decorticate the facet joint.

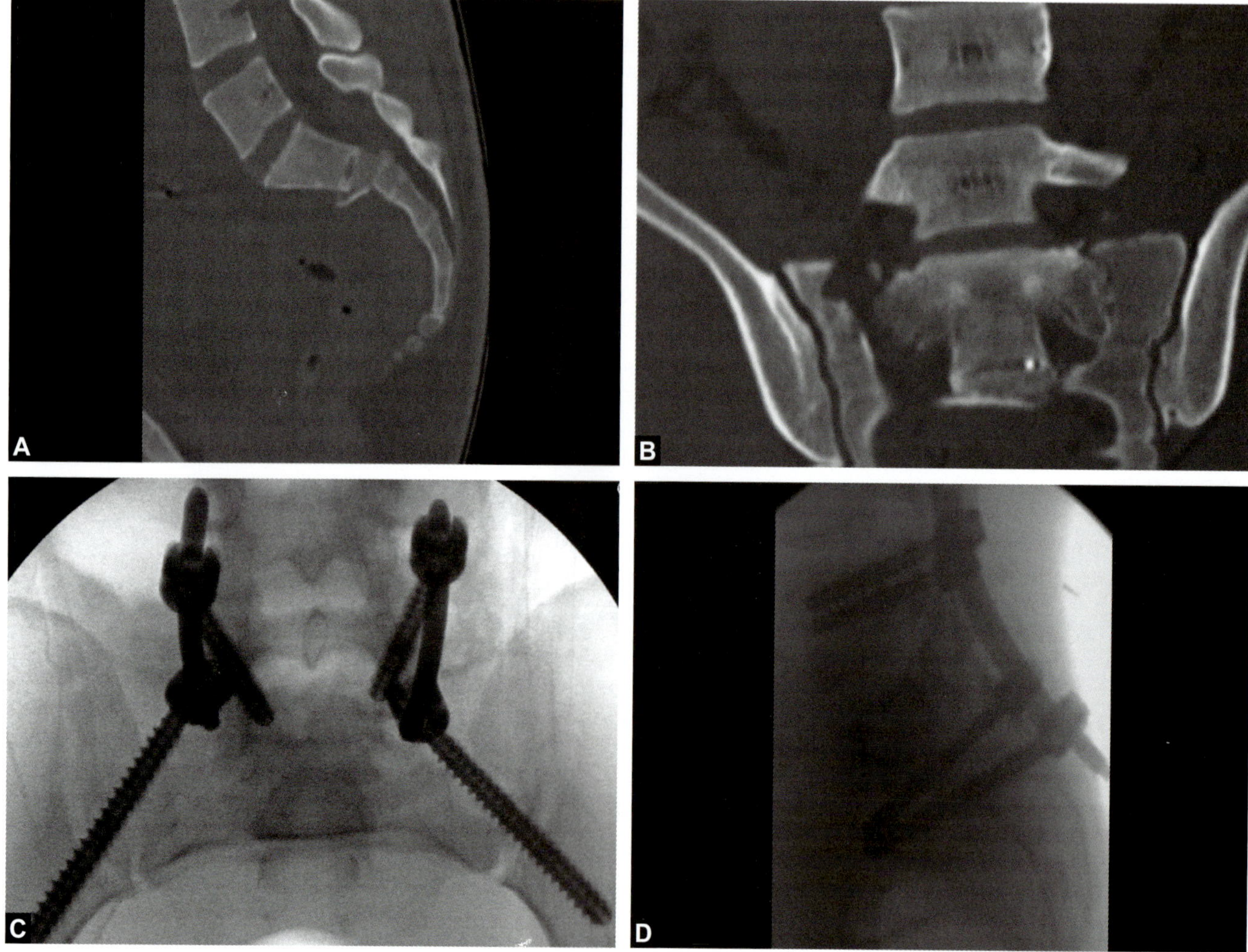

Figs. 15.2A to D: Patient who presented to the trauma bay after a high-speed motor vehicle accident and had multiple injuries including an H-type sacral fracture (A and B). He incurred significant abrasions near a traditional open surgical incision for lumbopelvic fixation. Thus, the sacral fracture was managed with percutaneous pedicle screw of L5 and iliac screw placement (C and D).

- Hemodynamically unstable patients or patients with multiorgan system injuries can benefit from percutaneous pedicle screw placement for initial stabilization (Figs. 15.3A to D).
  - After resuscitation, the patient may return to the operating room for a fusion procedure.

Pitfalls

- Pedicle screw fixation alone is not sufficient. Adjunct fusion procedures are required to prevent failure of instrumentation with cyclical loading.
- In a trauma setting preoperative planning demands the same meticulous assessment as in any other situation avoid pedicle screw misplacement (Figs. 15.4A and B).

SURGICAL TECHNIQUES

Posterior Percutaneous Pedicle Screw Fixation

- Multiple techniques are available for safe and effective pedicle screw placement.
  - Biplanar fluoroscopy
  - Image-guided navigation
  - Magerl (or 'owl's eye') technique

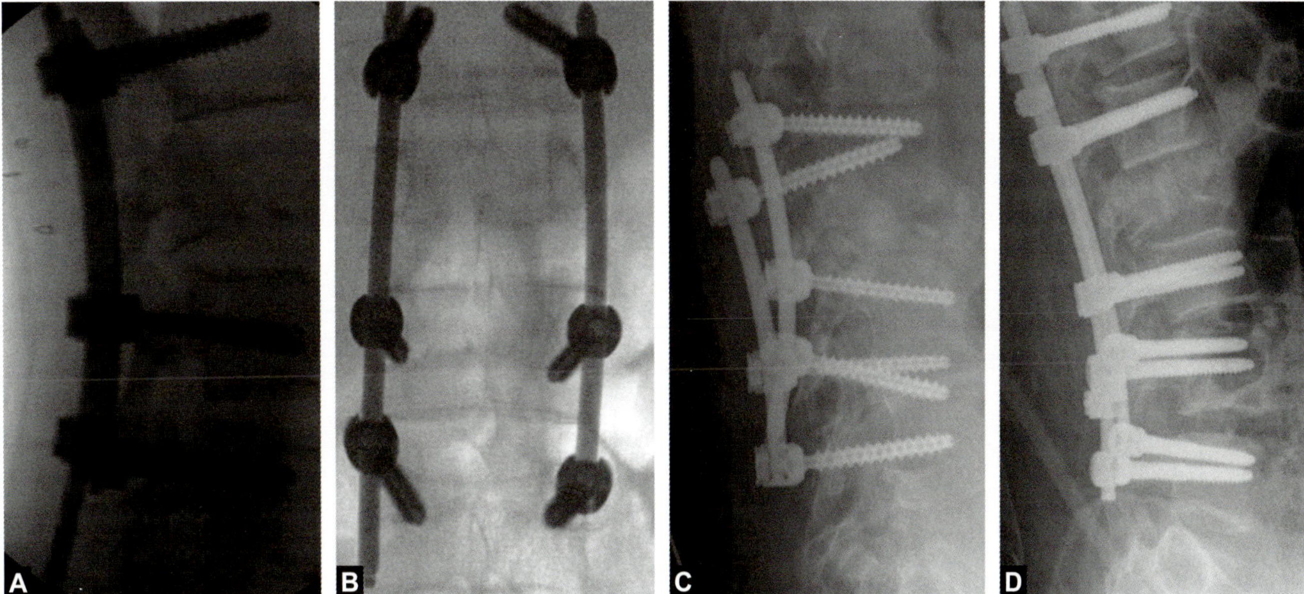

Figs. 15.3A to D: Polytrauma patient who presented with multiple injuries including an L2 burst fracture. Initial management involved percutaneous pedicle screw placement for damage-control spine stabilization (A and B). After a prolonged hospital stay, the spinal construct lost fixation (C). The spinal fixation was converted to an open technique with a construct from T12–L5 (D).

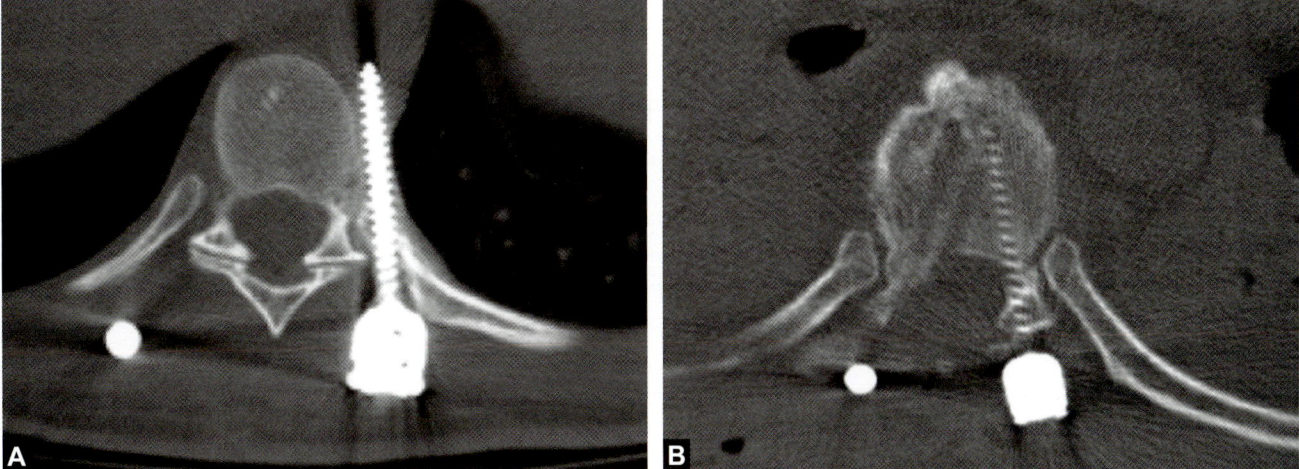

Figs. 15.4A and B: Pedicle screw misplacement: (A) Lateral placement of percutaneous screw: the screw length is too long and abuts the aorta. (B) Medial placement of the percutaneous screw. The screw tract demonstrates that the canal was violated. The patient developed a temporary neurologic deficit that resolved after screw removal and a laminectomy.

- True AP targeting
  - Deciding which technique to utilize depends upon the surgeon's preference and experience.
  - If intraoperative fluoroscopy is unable to provide adequate visualization, the procedure should not be undertaken.
- This can occur in patients with obesity, severely deformed anatomy, or osteopenia.
- Access to more advanced intraoperative imaging may be necessary [intraoperative CT (O-Arm)] or an open procedure should be performed.

ROD PLACEMENT

- After placement of the necessary pedicle screws, a properly sized and contoured rod is passed in a cranial to caudal direction.
  - Technically sound pedicle screw placement will facilitate the rod insertion.
    - The depth of the screw heads should be similar and the top of the screw extensions should demonstrate a smooth transition.
- A two-handed technique will provide appropriate sensory feedback to the surgeon during rod placement.
  - The dominant hand should be on the rod holder while the other hand adjusts the orientation of the rod extensions.

Pearls

- A minimally invasive lateral corpectomy and cage placement avoids the need for an access surgeon.

Pitfalls

- For lumbar fractures, a transpsoas approach can be associated with postoperative lower extremity pain or weakness from injury to the lumbar plexus and/or the psoas muscle.

MINIMALLY INVASIVE LATERAL CORPECTOMY AND CAGE PLACEMENT

- This minimally invasive approach can provide adequate exposure if decompression and reconstruction of the anterior column is indicated.
- Care must be taken to avoid further neurological compromise when placing the patient into a decubitus lateral position.
  - Initial posterior fixation with percutaneous pedicle screw placement can help stabilize the spine prior to lateral decubitus positioning.

CONCLUSION

- A trauma patient may benefit from a minimally invasive spinal stabilization by virtue of the reduced operative time, blood loss, and postoperative pain. In addition, minimally invasive procedures are associated with a lower infection rate and shorter recovery time.[1,4]
- Minimally invasive spinal stabilization with percutaneous screws is an appropriate treatment option for unstable thoracolumbar spine fractures and for patients with life-threatening multisystem injuries.[1,2]
- Pedicle screw fixation without concomitant fusion for stable thoracolumbar burst fractures provides similar clinical and radiographic outcomes as those who undergo a concurrent posterolateral fusion.[4] However, the role for surgical treatment in stable burst fractures remains controversial.
- There are limited reports on the utilization of percutaneous pedicle screw fixation for the treatment of thoracolumbar fractures. For this reason, some authors have raised concerns regarding the effectiveness of this minimally invasive technique in correcting the spinal deformity and achieving a bony fusion.[5]

Pearls

- If there is no discoligamentous injury associated with the spinal fracture, the instrumentation can be removed after the bone heals.

Controversies

- The utilization of bone graft is not required in fractures where the instability is completely bone related.

REFERENCES

1. Banagan K, Ludwig SC. Thoracolumbar spine trauma: when damage control minimally invasive spine surgery is an option. Semin Spine Surg. 2012;24:221-5.
2. Court C, Vincent C. Percutaneous fixation of thoracolumbar fractures: current concepts. Orthop Traumatol Surg Res: OTSR 2012;98:900-9.

3. Rampersaud YR, Annand N, Dekutoski MB. Use of minimally invasive surgical techniques in the management of thoracolumbar trauma—current concepts. Spine. 2006;32:S96-102.
4. Dai LY, Jiang LS, Jiang SD. Posterior short-segment fixation with or without fusion for thoracolumbar burst fractures. a five to seven-year prospective randomized study. The J Bone Joint Surgery Am. 2009;91:1033-41.
5. Barbagallo GMV, Yoder E, Dettori JR, Albanese V. Percutaneous minimally invasive versus open spine surgery in the treatment of fractures of the thoracolumbar junction—a comparative effectiveness review. Evid Based Spine Care J. 2012;3:43-9.

REFERENCE SUMMARY

1. Banagan K, Ludwig SC. Thoracolumbar Spine Trauma: When damage control minimally invasive spine surgery is an option. Seminars in Spine Surgery 2012;24:221-5.
   Summary: The authors discuss the role of minimally invasive spine surgery for the treatment of spinal trauma. In the setting of a polytrauma patient with multiple organ system injuries, a minimally invasive temporizing percutaneous pedicle screw fixation is an effective option for early stabilization.
2. Court C, Vincent C. Percutaneous fixation of thoracolumbar fractures: current concepts. Orthopaedics & Traumatology, Surgery & Research: OTSR. 2012;98:900-909.
   Summary: A literature review on the indications and limitations of minimally invasive techniques for the treatment of thoracolumbar fractures. The authors discuss the scenarios amenable to percutaneous fixation alone and in combination with other procedures including a cement augmentation and an open or minimally invasive decompression and fusion.
3. Rampersaud YR, Annand N, Dekutoski MB. Use of minimally invasive surgical techniques in the management of thoracolumbar trauma—current concepts. Spine. 2006;32:S96-S102.
   Summary: A literature review discussing the rationale, clinical applications, outcomes, and limitation of minimally invasive techniques for thoracolumbar spine trauma. The authors concluded that the indications of a minimally invasive technique for the treatment of a thoracolumbar fracture and the associated technologies are still evolving, but that the current literature is encouraging.
4. Dai LY, Jiang LS, Jiang SD. Posterior short-segment fixation with or without fusion for thoracolumbar burst fractures. a five to seven-year prospective randomized study. The Journal of Bone and Joint Surgery American volume 2009;91:1033-41.
   Summary: A randomized controlled trial of 73 patients who underwent a posterior pedicle screw instrumentation with and without concurrent posterolateral fusion for Denis type-B burst fractures and a load-shearing score ≤ 6. The operative time and blood loss were significantly lower in the non-fusion groups. However, at 5 years of follow-up, there were no differences with regards to the radiographic and clinical outcomes between the two cohorts.
5. Barbagallo GMV, Yoder E, Dettori JR, Albanese V. Percutaneous minimally invasive versus open spine surgery in the treatment of fractures of the thoracolumbar junction—a comparative effectiveness review. Evid Based Spine Care J 2012;3:43-49.
   Summary: A literature review comparing the effectiveness and safety of percutaneous versus open surgery for thoracolumbar fractures. The authors reported that percutaneous fixation techniques for thoracolumbar fractures are associated with reduced postoperative pain, blood loss, and hospital stay. However, the authors concluded that the limited data regarding the minimally invasive techniques for the management of spinal trauma warrant further studies to validate the efficacy of percutaneous techniques in correcting spinal deformity and achieving a bony fusion.

Chapter

16

Minimally Invasive Bone Grafts and Osteobiologics

Sreeharsha V Nandyala, Kris B Siemionow, Kern Singh

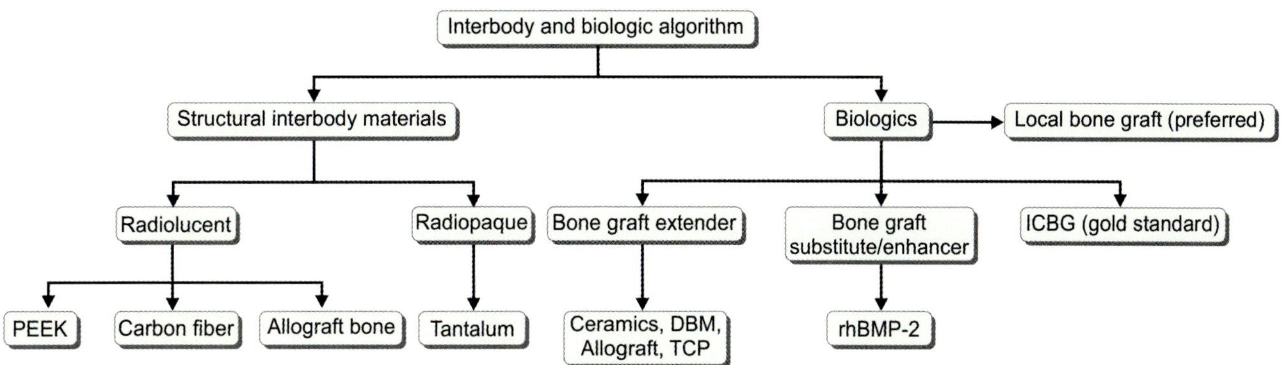

CASE VIGNETTE

A 57-year-old man who underwent an L5–S1 transforaminal interbody fusion (TLIF) 2 years ago presents with recurrent back and lower extremity pain. On examination, the patient demonstrates diminished sensation over the lateral aspect of the ankles and inability to walk on his toes. The Achilles tendon reflex is also diminished on the right. Imaging studies confirm an L5–S1 pseudarthrosis with graft migration. The patient is scheduled for a revision L5–S1 fusion either through a mini-open anterior approach or a minimally invasive (MIS) posterolateral fusion.

PRINCIPLES OF LUMBAR INTERBODY FUSION

- The goals of a lumbar interbody fusion (LIF) include a solid, stable, and load-sustaining arthrodesis while maintaining the disc height and restoring sagittal plane alignment.
- Methodical and thorough preparation of the bony host site (i.e. facet joints, vertebral endplates) is essential to potentiate arthrodesis with the bone graft.
- A MIS LIF is associated with a limited exposure, a scarcity of local bone graft, and a reduced surface area to promote a bony fusion. For this reason, there is a greater demand for safe and effective biologics to help promote a successful fusion.

Pearls

- The most sensitive diagnostic test for assessing fusion is a CT scan with axial, sagittal, and coronal reconstructions.

- The ideal bone graft is characterized by having osteoinductive, osteoconductive, and osteogenic properties while minimizing local tissue reactions, disease transmission, and patient morbidity (harvest site).

IMPLANT CHARACTERISTICS THAT PROMOTE SPINAL FUSION

Structural Implant Designs

- Cage geometry (wedge shaped, rectangular, banana shaped), size, and positioning play a significant role in restoring disc height and sagittal alignment.
  - These implants provide initial distraction, segmental stability, and support during axial loading.
    - Wedge-shaped cages increase lordosis (when placed anteriorly in the disc space) and can be utilized for restoring sagittal alignment from a posterior approach.
- Structural implants eliminate the need to harvest large autologous bone grafts, thereby avoiding bone graft harvest morbidity.
- Stackable and expandable cages can be utilized for reconstruction of the anterior column through an anterior or lateral approach.
  - Cages can be utilized in the setting of tumors, infection, trauma, or degenerative conditions.
  - Expandable cages can perform indirect foraminal decompression.
- Insertion devices have evolved to guide the implant into the appropriate location in the interbody space from various angles and trajectories.
  - A hinge component is often incorporated in the implant design that allows the cage to be guided into an anterior-central position within the disc space through a MIS posterior approach.

Interbody Spacers

- Allograft spacers
  - Cortical bone grafts are shaped into interbody spacers, which act as an osteoconductive scaffold that allow the host endplates to incorporate into the cadaveric bone.
  - Allograft spacers provide initial mechanical and structural support, which is an advantage when promoting arthrodesis.
  - These implants are often more brittle than synthetic grafts and can fracture during the press fit placement.
  - In addition, cortical allograft spacers have a relatively high Young's modulus, which increases the risk for implant subsidence when compared with synthetic implants.
- Polyetheretherketone spacers (PEEK) (Figs. 16.1A and B)
  - The PEEK spacers design incorporates a graft window for the placement of bone autografts or biologic substitutes to promote arthrodesis.
  - These spacers have a similar modulus of elasticity to that of cancellous bone, which allow axial load transfer onto the bone graft.

Pearls

- A titanium cage can lead to subsidence, stress shielding, and obscures the bone graft on plain radiographs. Titanium is not typically utilized in this setting because of the modulus mismatch and radioopacity.

Pitfalls

- A successful MIS approach relies upon both direct and indirect decompression of the neural elements. Cage subsidence can have significant clinical consequences.

Pearls

- The largest possible PEEK spacer should be utilized to reduce the risk of implant subsidence.

Pitfalls

- Although both PEEK and carbon fiber cages have demonstrated satisfactory clinical and radiographic outcomes, no prospective clinical study has directly compared these two implants.

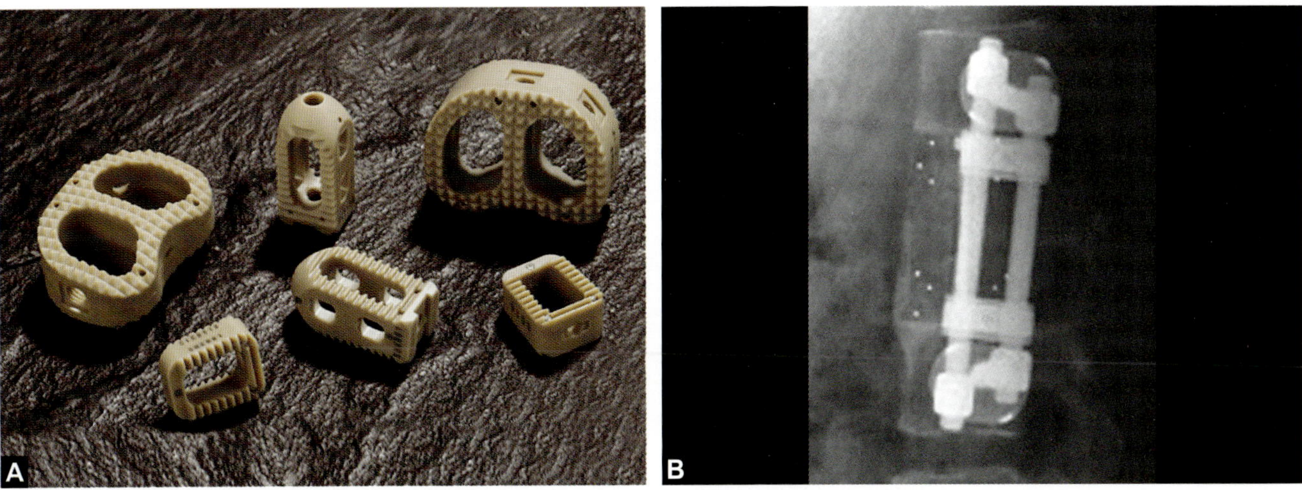

Figs. 16.1A and B: (A) PEEK spacers. (B) A PEEK expandable corpectomy cage has been utilized for spinal reconstruction. There is evidence of bone growth through the cage.

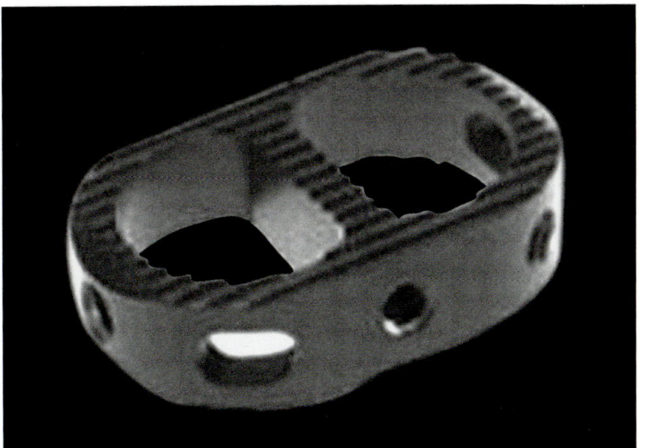

Fig. 16.2: Carbon fiber reinforced polymer cages.

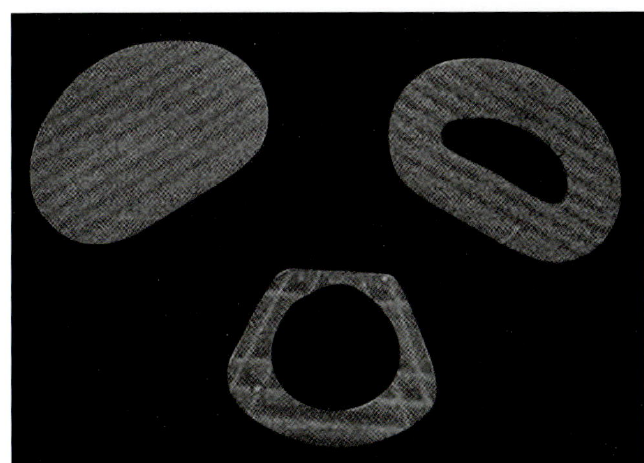

Fig. 16.3: Porous tantalum implants.

- In addition, the radiolucency of PEEK implants facilitates the evaluation of fusion on plain radiographs and computed tomography (CT).
- In contrast to allografts, there is no concern for disease transmission and quality does not vary from implant to implant.
- PEEK spacers have no osteoinductive, osteogenic, or osteoconductive properties.

- Carbon fiber-enforced polymer cages (Fig. 16.2)
  - The cage design typically includes ridges or teeth that resist retropulsion.
  - The stiffness of these cages is five times greater than PEEK and more closely approximates the modulus of cortical bone.
  - Carbon fiber spacers can be stacked together to fill large defects while maintaining appropriate stress distribution onto the graft material.
- Porous tantalum (Fig. 16.3)
  - Tantalum is a trabecular metal that is approximately 70–80% porous with an average pore size of 400–500 μm.

- Its stiffness is similar to that of cancellous bone, which provides physiologic load transfer and a reduced stress shielding that results in the preservation of bone.
- Similar to the other interbody spacers, it provides primary stability and eliminates the need to harvest a large bone graft to fill significant defects.
- The implant design consists of a peripheral structure with a central cavity for placing graft material
- Tantalum implants are radiopaque and because of their metallic composition may significantly degrade CT and magnetic resonance imaging postoperatively.

BONE GRAFTS

Bone Graft Characteristics

- Osteoinduction—The recruitment and stimulation of pluripotential mesenchymal cells to differentiate into osteoblasts and osteoclasts. A true osteoinductive agent will promote bone formation in any tissue in the body.
- Osteoconduction—Structural scaffolding provided by a graft material that allows the proliferation and incorporation of new blood vessels and bone.
- Osteogenesis—The formation of osteoblasts directly from the existing mesenchymal cells within the graft.

Bone Autograft

- Types of bone autografts
  - Cortical—Provides immediate mechanical strength and support but has less osteoinductive and osteoconductive properties than cancellous bone
  - Cancellous—Offers osteoinductive and osteoconductive properties to the graft site but has diminished structural support
  - Corticocancellous—Provides both mechanical support with osteoinductive and osteoconductive properties, which fulfills the criteria for an ideal bone graft
    - Iliac crest bone graft (ICBG) is considered the gold standard to which other biologics are compared.
- The risk of disease transmission and immune reactions is significantly reduced with the utilization of synthetic grafts.
- Despite its obvious advantages, bone autografts have a limited supply and may be associated with significant donor site morbidity (i.e. pain, paresthesia, infection).
- Local bone autograft (obtained from morselized lamina during the exposure) may be utilized in the intervertebral space.
  - Local bone graft does not require a separate harvest site, which reduces surgical time and eliminates the risk of harvest site morbidity.
  - In a MIS approach, the amount of local bone autograft may be insufficient.

Local autograft pitfalls

- Local bone autograft may not provide sufficient graft material, especially for revision cases (previous laminectomy)

- A suction canister can be utilized to trap the "bone dust" that is generated from the burr during the MIS decompression. The viability of this bone is poorly understood. Regardless, the graft obtained can serve as a bulking agent (osteoconductive scaffold with minimal osteoinductive properties)
- Effective bone graft substitutes and extenders (cadaveric or synthetic) are therefore essential to achieve fusion.

BONE GRAFT SUBSTITUTES AND OSTEOBIOLOGICS

- Bone allografts
  - Bone allografts are readily available and are not associated with autograft harvest site morbidity.
  - Although small, there is a risk of disease transmission and host immune reaction.
  - The preparation of most bone allografts includes tissue freezing, freeze-drying, and gamma radiation.
    - This sterilization process reduces the risk of disease transmission and host immune response at the expense of loosing osteoinductive capabilities.
    - Processing method may affect the structural properties of the graft.
  - Allografts alone can provide a solid scaffold for bony in-growth (osteoconductive).
  - The combination of bone allografts with bone autografts or growth factors adds the osteoinductive properties required to enhance fusion.
- Synthetic bone grafts
  - Synthetic bone grafts include ceramics, bioglass, silicates, or collagen. These synthetic grafts form a scaffold for bony in-growth.
  - The advantages of a synthetic bone graft lie in its inert biocompatible, osteoconductive properties, and abundant availability.
  - The rate of reabsorption of some materials precludes their utilization in spine surgery.
    - Calcium sulfate—Resorbs in 4–12 weeks
    - Calcium phosphate—Resorbs in 26–86 weeks
    - Hydroxyapatite—Resorbs in 1–5 years
  - Synthetic bone grafts should only be utilized in combination with other bone grafts or substitutes to promote fusion.
- Demineralized bone matrix (DBM)
  - This unique allograft is produced by acid extraction of cortical bone, which results in removal of the mineral contents but leaves behind growth factors (bone morphogenetic protein, BMP) and proteins.
    - DBM is available in a variety of presentations including freeze-dried powder, granules, gel, putty, and chips
    - DBM contains type 1 collagen, which provides an osteoconductive scaffold for bony in-growth. Depending on its preparation and presentation, DBM will provide a different degree of osteoinductive potency.

DBM Pitfalls

- DBM preparation, and thus BMP concentration, differs between commercial companies. In addition, large batches from the same manufacturer may also contain different concentrations of BMP.

- DBM is generally utilized as an adjunct to other grafting material (autografts) or as a graft extender, since it provides little to no mechanical and structural properties.
- Growth factors—Bone morphogenetic proteins
  - BMPs help regulate differentiation, maturation, and proliferation of mesenchymal precursor cells into osteogenic and chondrogenic cells.
  - BMP requires the utilization of a carrier matrix to hold the growth factor at the graft site and prevent extravasation to adjacent tissues.
  - There are two commercially available forms of BMP.
    - INFUSE (rhBMP-2)—FDA approved for ALIF with titanium cage
    - OP-1 (rhBMP-7)
  - Controversies surrounding BMP include:
    - An extensive literature and industry data review by an independent group demonstrated that the currently published literature is biased with an underreporting of complications.[2,3]
    - A theoretically increased risk for carcinogenesis is associated with the utilization of BMP but definitive evidence is lacking.
    - Other complications associated with BMP include anterior neck swelling, osteolysis, retrograde ejaculation, urinary retention, radiculitis, and seroma formation.

Contraindications to BMP

- Pregnancy
- History of cancer
- Skeletal immaturity
- History of bone tumors

Pearls

- Some surgeons have reported a reduced potential for local postoperative complications (radiculitis, ectopic bone formation, and osteolysis) by placing barriers such as fibrin glue, duraseal, or bone wax at the annulotomy site.

CONCLUSION

- In the published literature, there is significant controversy regarding the utilization of BMP as a substitute for ICBG. While some meta-analyses have demonstrated similar arthrodesis rates between BMP and ICBG,[2] there are potential causes for concern regarding complications that may arise from improper dosing.[1]
- Multiple BMP-related adverse events have been described including retrograde ejaculation, ectopic bone formation, and cancer. However, the majority of the published literature has significant statistical limitations, which preclude any definitive conclusion regarding the efficacy and safety of BMP utilization.[1-3]
- The utilization of BMP in the setting of an MIS TLIF may be associated with a greater arthrodesis rate and a reduced potential for pseudarthrosis and reoperation when compared with an adjuvant silicate-substituted calcium phosphate (Actifuse).[4]
- PEEK cages are safe and effective synthetic spacers for MIS lumbar fusion. The reported implant subsidence rate is 14.3%, but only 2.1% of patients become symptomatic. Adequate endplate preparation, a clear understanding of the regional anatomy, the utilization of a wide implant and adequate implant positioning can help mitigate the risk for implant subsidence.[5]

REFERENCES

1. Singh K, Ahmadinia K, Park DK, et al. Complications of spinal fusion with utilization of bone morphogenetic protein: a systematic review of the literature. Spine J. 2013;39(1):91-101.

2. Simmonds MC, Brown JV, Heirs MK, et al. Safety and effectiveness of recombinant human bone morphogenetic protein-2 for spinal fusion. Ann Intern Med. 2013;158:877-89.
3. Fu R, Selph S, McDonagh M, et al. Effectiveness and harms of recombinant human bone morphogenetic protein-2 in spine fusion: a systematic review and meta-analysis. Ann Intern Med. 2013;158:890-902.
4. Nandyala SV, Marquez-Lara A, Fineberg SJ, Pelton M, Singh K. A prospective, randomized, controlled trial of silicate substituted calcium phosphate versus rhBMP-2 in a minimally invasive transforaminal lumbar interbody fusion. Spine. (Phila Pa 1976).2014;39:185-91.
5. Le TV, Baaj AA, Dakwar E, et al. Subsidence of polyetheretherketone intervertebral cages in minimally invasive lateral retroperitoneal transpsoas lumbar interbody fusion. Spine (Phila Pa 1976). 2012;37:1268-73.

REFERENCE SUMMARY

1. Singh K, Ahmadinia K, Park DK, Nandyala SV, Marquez-Lara A, Patel AA, Fineberg SJ. Complications of spinal fusion with utilization of bone morphogenetic protein: a systematic review of the literature. The Spine Journal. 2013;39(1):91-101.
   Summary: A systematic review to identify the types of complications associated with the utilization of bone morphogenetic protein (BMP) in cervical and lumbar spine surgery. The pseudarthrosis rates were significantly lower with the utilization of BMP in all procedures except for PLIF/TLIFs. The only statistically significant adverse complication rate was retrograde ejaculation in the ALIF population. The authors concluded that despite the increased awareness of complications associated with BMP, the complication rates are low and are specific to the spinal level.
2. Simmonds MC, Brown JV, Heirs MK, Higgins JP, Mannion RJ, Rodgers MA, Stewart LA. Safety and effectiveness of recombinant human bone morphogenetic protein-2 for spinal fusion. Ann Intern Med. 2013;158:877-89.
   Summary: A review of the industry sponsored randomized, controlled trials of rhBMP-2 versus iliac crest bone graft (ICBG) in spinal fusion surgery. The authors concluded that at 24 months, rhBMP-2 was associated with an increased fusion rate and early postsurgical pain compared with ICBG. In addition, the evidence correlating carcinogenesis with rhBMP-2 is inconclusive.
3. Fu R, Selph S, McDonagh M, Peterson K, Tiwari A, Chou R, Helfand M. Effectiveness and harms of recombinant human bone morphogenetic protein-2 in spine fusion: a systematic review and meta-analysis. Ann Intern Med 2013;158:890-902.
   Summary: An independent assessment of the effectiveness and harms of rhBMP-2 utilization for spinal fusion and the reporting bias among the industry-sponsored journal publications. After reviewing the available industry sponsored, randomized, controlled trials, the authors reported that the early rhBMP-2-related publications misrepresented the effectiveness and harms through selective reporting, duplicate publication, and underreporting. The authors concluded that for spinal fusion, rhBMP-2 has no proven clinical advantage over bone graft and is likely associated with important harms.
4. Nandyala SV, Marquez-Lara A, Fineberg SJ, Pelton M, Singh K. A prospective, randomized, controlled trial of silicate substituted calcium phosphate versus rhBMP-2 in a minimally invasive transforaminal lumbar interbody fusion. Spine. (Phila Pa 1976).2014;39:185-91.
   Summary: A prospective, randomized, controlled trial comparing the arthrodesis rates between patients undergoing a primary single-level minimally invasive TLIF with either Actifuse or bone morphogenetic protein (rhBMP-2). At 1-year follow-up, the fusion rates in the BMP cohort were significantly greater when compared with the Actifuse-treated group (92% vs 65%).

5. Le TV, Baaj AA, Dakwar E, et al. Subsidence of polyetheretherketone intervertebral cages in minimally invasive lateral retroperitoneal transpsoas lumbar interbody fusion. Spine (Phila Pa 1976) 2012;37:1268-73.
Summary: A retrospective review of 140 patients who underwent a minimally invasive lateral retroperitoneal lumbar interbody fusion utilizing a polyetheretherketone (PEEK) cage. The implant subsidence rate was 14.3% but only 2.1% were clinically significant. The authors concluded that the wider intervertebral cages reduced the risk for implant subsidence and promoted arthrodesis.

Index

Note: Page numbers followed by *f* and *fc* refer to Figure and Flowchart, respectively.

G

H

I

J

K

L

M

N

O

P

Q

R

S

T

U

V

W

Withdrawn